Small Animal Dental Procedures
for Veterinary Technicians and Nurses

Small Animal Dental Procedures
for Veterinary Technicians and Nurses

Second Edition

Edited by

Jeanne R. Perrone, MS, CVT, VTS (Dentistry)
VT Dental Training
Plant City, FL, USA

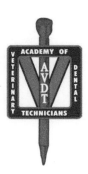

WILEY Blackwell

Registered Office
John Wiley & Sons, Inc., 111 River Street, Hoboken, NJ 07030, USA

Editorial Office
111 River Street, Hoboken, NJ 07030, USA

For details of our global editorial offices, customer services, and more information about Wiley products visit us at www.wiley.com.

Wiley also publishes its books in a variety of electronic formats and by print-on-demand. Some content that appears in standard print versions of this book may not be available in other formats.

Library of Congress Cataloging-in-Publication Data

Names: Perrone, Jeanne R., editor.
Title: Small animal dental procedures for veterinary technicians and nurses / edited by Jeanne R. Perrone.
Description: Second edition. | Hoboken, NJ : Wiley-Blackwell, [2021] | Includes bibliographical references and index.
Identifiers: LCCN 2020017966 (print) | LCCN 2020017967 (ebook) | ISBN 9781119451839 (paperback) | ISBN 9781119451846 (adobe pdf) | ISBN 9781119451853 (epub)
Subjects: MESH: Dental Care–veterinary | Pets | Animals, Exotic | Animal Technicians
Classification: LCC SF867 (print) | LCC SF867 (ebook) | NLM SF 867 | DDC 636.089/76–dc23
LC record available at https://lccn.loc.gov/2020017966
LC ebook record available at https://lccn.loc.gov/2020017967

Cover Design: Wiley
Cover Image: Courtesy of Jeanne R. Perrone

Set in 10/12pt Sabon by SPi Global, Pondicherry, India

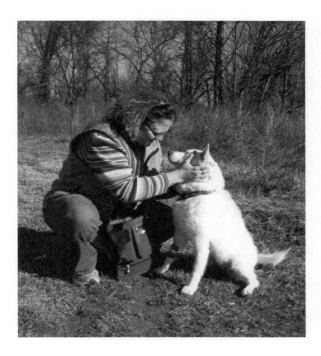

To my dad, Frank, who taught me responsibility and the value of providing quality medicine

To my mom, Priscilla, who taught me compassion and giving

To my stepmom, Lynn, who taught me how to be resourceful

To my sister, Zan, who taught me how to be independent

To my brother, Andy, who taught me never to give up

To my sister-in-law, Lucy, who taught me that all challenges can be overcome with grace

To my niece, Jasmine, who taught me maturity

To my nephew, Jordan, who taught me spirit and bravery

To my best friend and confidant, Lisa, for over 30 years of being a part of my life

To the members of the AVDT who have brought me love and laughter since the year 2000

To all the veterinary technicians, veterinary assistants, veterinarians, and veterinary dentists I have been blessed to work with for making me into the technician I am today

To my Tony, who constantly teaches this Italian girl how to be a little more Puerto Rican

To my pets and patients, past and present, my source of love and acceptance

Lastly, to Luna, our model for the medical diagrams in Chapter 1 and a former patient of mine. I received word from her mom and our artist, Brenda Gregory, that she passed away from an inoperable tumor on December 29, 2011. Her mother, Brenda, is grateful that she will be immortalized in this book.

Contents

For materials available online only,
go to www.wiley.com/go/perrone/dental

Contributors

Benita Altier, LVT, VTS (Dentistry)
Pawsitive Dental Education, LLC
Easton, WA, USA

Mary Berg, BS, RLATG, RVT, VTS
(Dentistry)
Beyond the Crown Veterinary Dental
Education
Lawrence, KS, USA

Laurel Bird, CVT, VTS (Dentistry)
Animal Emergency and Referral Center
of MN
Menomonie, WI, USA

Jennifer Crawford, LVT, VTS
(Dentistry)
East Lansing, MI, USA

Patricia Dominguez, LVT, VTS (Dentistry)
Briarwood, NY, USA

Candice Hoerner, CVT, VTS (Dentistry)
Big Sky Veterinary Dentistry Education
Whitefish, MT, USA

Gerianne Holzman, CVT, VTS
(Dentistry-Retired)
UW Veterinary Care Emerita
University of Wisconsin
Middleton, WI, USA

Kathy Istace, CVT, VTS (Dentistry)
Mayfield Veterinary Hospital
Edmonton, AB, Canada

Billie Jean (Jeannie) Losey, RVT, VTS
(Dentistry)
NCSU Health and Wellness Center –
Dentistry
Raleigh, NC, USA

Patricia A. March, RVT, VTS
(Dentistry)
Animal Dental Center
Towson, MD, USA

Julie McMahon, LVT, VTS (Dentistry)
Sierra Veterinary Specialists
Reno, NV, USA

Annie Mills, LVT, VTS (Dentistry)
Florida Veterinary Dentistry and Oral
Surgery
Debary, FL, USA

Judy Ozier, CVT, VTS
(Dentistry-Retired)
Sullivan, IL, USA

Jeanne R. Perrone, MS, CVT, VTS
(Dentistry)
VT Dental Training
Plant City, FL, USA

Sara Sharp, CVT, VTS (Dentistry)
Bel Rae Institute
Denver, CO, USA

Foreword

In the year 2000, a group of veterinary technicians with a passion for veterinary dentistry began an arduous journey. Their vision was to form a dental specialty organization for technicians who wish to excel in the field. The Academy of Veterinary Dental Technicians (AVDT) was formed. Over the next several years, the organizing committee succeeded in writing a constitution and an exam, which is given annually to qualified candidates. AVDT also had to meet specific guidelines for technicians seeking to become Veterinary Technician Specialists. Today AVDT is recognized by both the National Association of Veterinary Technicians in America (NAVTA) and the American Veterinary Dental College (AVDC).

Since the beginning, ADVT has provided an avenue for technicians and assistants involved with dentistry to grow and learn together. The idea for this book has evolved over time. All of the existing written material for veterinary dentistry has been provided by the veterinarians in the field. AVDT has chosen to use our pool of very knowledgeable and qualified veterinary technician specialists to write a dental book by technicians specifically for the use of other technicians, assistants, and students.

This book is designed to be a learning tool to increase skill levels and understanding of various dental procedures. Basic dental skills, such as doing a complete prophylaxis, charting teeth, and taking diagnostic radiographs, are just a few examples of essential tasks that we should to able to perform competently. Additionally, it is necessary to have the knowledge of more complex dental procedures.

Increasing our levels of competence yields many tangible benefits to us all. In addition to achieving pride in our accomplishments, we become more valuable members of the veterinary dental health care team. Our increased knowledge allows us to pursue job opportunities with potential monetary increase. We will also establish a necessary foundation to pursue our professional challenges in a knowledgeable manner.

It is our hope that you will find this book to be a good reference guide, a resource to find specific dental information that will help make your dental experiences less intimidating, and a resource for you to hone your skills and tweak areas that need improvement. Remember that we all have our patients' best interests in mind and our ultimate goal is to provide them with good oral health through our best efforts.

Judy Ozier, CVT, VTS (Dentistry Retired)

Foreword from Academy of Veterinary Dental Technicians

The Academy of Veterinary Dental Technicians (AVDT) has partnered with Wiley to bring this text to you to encourage the education and training of veterinary technicians and nurses. It is a comprehensive text that will supply detailed knowledge to the reader of how to prevent, identify, and treat common oral conditions. This expanded second edition will supply additional information in order for the veterinary team to provide the highest standard of dental care to our patients.

I am extremely proud of the authors' willingness to review and expand the chapters within the covers of this book. Veterinary dentistry is continually evolving, and we feel it is paramount to remain current within our profession. Our editor has spent countless hours reviewing this text to provide the readers with a high-quality resource for veterinary dentistry.

The AVDT is a group of technicians who have completed the rigorous requirements to become a Veterinary Technician Specialist (VTS) in Dentistry and are recognized by the National Association of Veterinary Technicians in America (NAVTA). These technicians have attained a higher level of recognition and advanced knowledge and skills in the field of dentistry. The members of the AVDT are considered experts in the field of dentistry and enjoy sharing their knowledge within the veterinary team and advancing the quality of care for our patients.

This book could not have been completed without the encouragement and support from the AVDT members and their families, the American Veterinary Dental College (AVDC), and The Foundation of Veterinary Dentistry. Thank you for making this project possible.

Candice Hoerner, CVT, VTS (Dentistry)
President, AVDT

Preface

With the upsurge in dental education available for veterinary technicians at the regional, state, and national levels, I am excited to provide the second edition of this text written for technicians by technicians.

The text is divided into 10 chapters, covering all branches of dentistry that the veterinary technician could encounter in practice. The contributors also touch upon the role of the veterinary technician, stressing the importance of connecting to the owner professionally using their dentistry knowledge. Professionalism is gained through education and experience.

This book is geared for technician students, working technicians, and technicians who are pursuing their specialty certification in dentistry. In keeping with changes in technology, the book has two components: the book and the website. The website component was added for two reasons: (1) there is sufficient space to store the large number of photographs and drawings that could not fit in the book and (2) it provides the reader with an extra educational experience using a project or a quiz based on the chapter. As requested by many of our reviewers, we have added video content to some of the chapters. These videos can be found in the web section of the book.

Acknowledgments

We would like to thank the following individuals and institutions:

University of Wisconsin Veterinary Medical Teaching Hospital
Patricia Dominguez, LVT, VTS (Dentistry)
IM3
Midmark Animal Health
Summit Hills Laboratories
Surgitel
Kristen Cooley, CVT, VTS (Anesthesia)
John Koehm, DVM, FAVD
Air Techniques Inc.
American Veterinary Dental College
Theresa Gabel, CVT
Ira Luskin, DVM, DAVDC
North Carolina State University
Skulls Unlimited International
Loic Legendre, DVM, FAVD, DAVDC, EVDC
Michael Fallon, DVM, PhD
Shipps Dental and Specialty Products
David Crossley, BVetMed
William Krug, DVM, DAVDC
Jean Dieden, DVM
Brian Hewitt, DVM, DAVDC
MAI Animal Health
Dentalaire
Gotham Veterinary Center
American Veterinary Dental College

Without their contributions, this book would not have come to be.

Jeanne R. Perrone

1 The Basics

Gerianne Holzman, CVT, VTS (Dentistry)

Learning Objectives

- Identify all anatomical sites and systems of the head, skull, and teeth
- Explain the relationship between structures in the oral cavity
- State the eruption timetable for primary and adult teeth
- Describe the stages of tooth development
- State the dental formula for the pediatric and adult dog and cat
- List and define oral directional terminology
- Define and perform both the anatomic and Triadan numbering systems used to count and identify teeth in the pediatric and adult dog and cat

Small Animal Dental Procedures for Veterinary Technicians and Nurses, Second Edition.
Edited by Jeanne R. Perrone.
© 2021 John Wiley & Sons, Inc. Published 2021 by John Wiley & Sons, Inc.

This comprehensive text on small animal dentistry meets the need for both novice and experienced veterinary technicians to advance their knowledge and explore new career paths. To learn advanced techniques, one needs to begin with the basics. This chapter discusses the anatomy of the skull and the teeth. With this knowledge, the veterinary technician learns the complex relationship between all structures surrounding the oral cavity. Dental disease, while generally thought of as a condition of the mouth, can also affect the nares, sinuses, and eyes.

Most mammals – including humans, dogs, and cats – have two sets of teeth in their lifetime: primary (or deciduous) and permanent (or secondary). Usually, the primary teeth exfoliate before the eruption of the permanent teeth. Malocclusions and dental disease can occur if this natural progression does not happen. (Two teeth should not occupy the same place at the same time.) Knowing the normal age of tooth eruption and the development of the tooth aids the veterinary technician in performing an oral exam.

In the mouth, the usual directional terminology of dorsal, ventral, medial, and lateral does not apply. The oral structures create a unique set of terms to determine location. Learning this specific terminology simplifies charting, surgical assisting, and explaining oral pathology.

Anatomy of the Skull[1]

Oral Cavity

The primary structures of the oral cavity consist of teeth, gingiva, tongue, soft palate, and hard palate. These vital organs of mastication and breathing can be involved with oral disease. Knowing what is normal helps in recognizing abnormalities.

Teeth[2]

Each species has a distinct dental formula. The dental formula is the number and types of teeth expected in a normal mouth. Dogs and cats have four types of teeth, each with separate purposes for eating and chewing. Domesticated animals, fed commercial diets, do not always use their teeth in the same manner as their wild ancestors. Incisors cut, pick up, and groom. Canines rip, tear, and hold. Premolars and molars grind food into a more digestible size (Figs. 1.1 and 1.2). Carnassials are the largest chewing teeth in the mouth. In both the dog and cat, they are the upper fourth premolar and the lower first molar.

Primary dental formula: canine (total 28)

■ Maxilla: incisors (6), canines (2), premolars (6), molars (0)
■ Mandible: incisors (6), canines (2), premolars (6), molars (0)

Permanent dental formula: canine (total 42)

■ Maxilla: incisors (6), canines (2), premolars (8), molars (4)
■ Mandible: incisors (6), canines (2), premolars (8), molars (6)

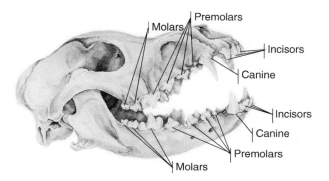

Figure 1.1 Canine skull showing permanent dentition (Illustration by Brenda Gregory).

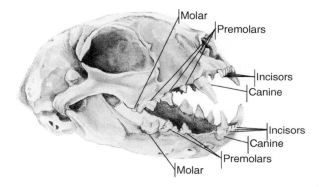

Figure 1.2 Feline skull showing permanent dentition (Illustration by Brenda Gregory).

Primary dental formula: feline (total 26)

- Maxilla: incisors (6), canines (2), premolars (6), molars (0)
- Mandible: incisors (6), canines (2), premolars (4) molars (0)

Permanent dental formula: feline (total 30)

- Maxilla: incisors (6), canines (2), premolars (6), molars (2)
- Mandible: incisors (6), canines (2), premolars (4), molars (2)

Dental formulae are often written as: canine (permanent): 2 × (I3/3, C1/1, P4/4, M2/3); and feline (permanent): 2 × (I3/3, C1/1, P3/2, M1/1). Anatomically, cats normally are missing their first upper premolars, first lower premolars, and second lower premolar teeth.

Gingiva[3]

The gingiva is the soft tissue surrounding and supporting the teeth. It also covers the alveolar bone supporting the teeth. Most often pink, the gingiva may be fully or partially pigmented. It should be glossy and smooth. Gingiva is modified epithelial and connective tissue. It divides into attached and unattached (or free) gingiva. Where the gingiva meets the rest of the oral mucosa of the lips is the mucogingival junction. Attached gingival tissue protects bone and tooth-supporting structures from infection, trauma, and periodontal disease. The junction between the free gingiva and the tooth is the gingival sulcus. Normal depth of this space is 3 mm in dogs and 1 mm in cats. If the depth of the sulcus is greater than normal, it indicates the presence of connective tissue loss known as a periodontal pocket. Pockets are often associated with gingivitis, an early form of periodontal disease.

Tongue

The tongue has four primary functions: to taste food, to lap up liquids, to form food into a bolus, and to aid in swallowing. Canines have a relatively smooth and over long tongue. Panting provides an efficient method for dogs to lower their body temperature. Feline tongues are rough due to the presence of firm, upright papillae, which aid in grooming and cleaning. The tongue can be pink or pigmented. In certain dog breeds (e.g., chow chows), the tongue is near to black. In dogs, a median groove is present on the dorsal surface. Hairs may grow in this groove. While aesthetically displeasing, they rarely cause injury.

The dorsal surface of the tongue contains papillae, some of which are specialized into taste buds. Different tastes and combinations – sweet, sour, bitter, and salty – are sensed over all surfaces of the tongue, not just in specific sections.

Specialized muscles and nerves of the tongue provide animals with the ability to drink fluids. A cat's tongue creates a "bowl" formation to allow it to scoop up water. In dogs, the tongue curls and twists water into the mouth. The tongue rolls food around the mouth forming a bolus or smooth round ball. With the aid of the tongue muscles, this bolus of food is then pushed to the back of the mouth and swallowed.

Hard and soft palate

The hard and soft palates comprise the "roof" of the oral cavity. The hard palate, created by the incisive, maxillary, and palatine bones, is covered by the soft tissue of the palatine rugae. The rugae, on each side of the palatine raphe (or midline), are symmetrical. Clefts or openings in the hard palate create direct access to the nasal cavity and sinuses. Surgical correction is appropriate for this genetic condition.

The incisive papilla located at the most rostral area of the hard palate is a raised round structure (Fig. 1.3). It aids in the senses of smell and taste and should not be confused with an oral mass. The soft palate is a continuation of the soft tissue overlying the hard palate. This movable fold of tissue connects the oral cavity to the pharynx. It is smooth and does not contain rugae.

Bones

The skull is composed of two sections: cranium and face. The cranium protects the brain and associated structures. The face comprises the bones of the oral, nasal, and ocular cavities. Bones provide the basic structure and support for blood vessels, muscles, tendons, all soft tissue structures, and teeth. Dogs and cats have three primary head shapes:

- Mesaticephalic or average (e.g., Labrador retriever [Fig. 1.4], German shepherd dog, domestic cat)

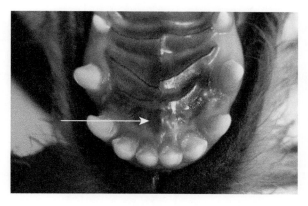

Figure 1.3 Incisive papilla in a canine (Courtesy of Jill Jecevicus).

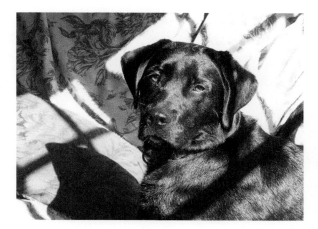

Figure 1.4 Mesaticephalic head shape: Labrador retriever.

- Brachycephalic or short-faced, resulting in crowded and rotated teeth (e.g., pug [Fig. 1.5], Persian cat, English bulldog)
- Dolichocephalic with a long narrow nose and face (e.g., Irish wolfhound, greyhound, Siamese cat [Fig. 1.6]).

Skull[4]

The primary bones of the cranium are:

- Frontal
- Parietal
- Interparietal
- Temporal
- Ethmoid
- Occipital
- Sphenoid

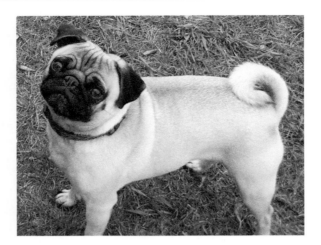

Figure 1.5 Brachycephalic head shape: pug.

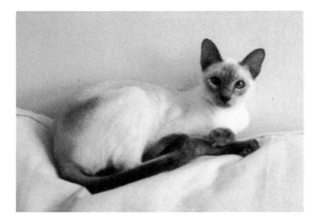

Figure 1.6 Dolichocephalic head shape: Siamese (Courtesy of Rebecca Johnson).

The facial bones consist of:

■ Lacrimal
■ Temporal process (includes zygomatic arch)
■ Nasal
■ Maxilla
■ Incisive
■ Pterygoid
■ Ventral nasal conchae
■ Mandible

The primary bones of the oral cavity are the mandibles and maxilla and the incisive. They support the teeth, attach to muscles, and provide protection to vessels and nerves. Within the mandible, maxilla, and incisive bones, the alveolus surrounds the tooth root and connects to the periodontal ligament (Figs. 1.7–1.9).

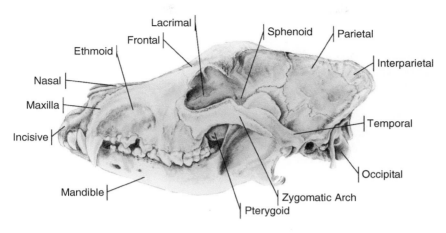

Figure 1.7 Lateral view of skull bones (Illustration by Brenda Gregory).

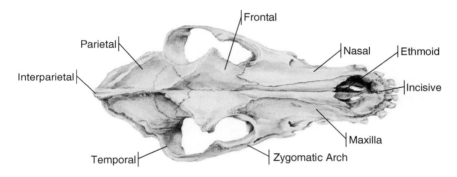

Figure 1.8 Dorsal view of skull bones (Illustration by Brenda Gregory).

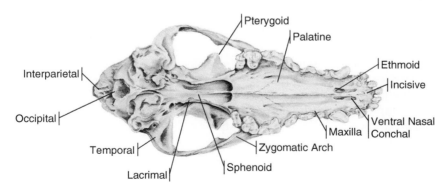

Figure 1.9 Palatine view of skull bones (Illustration by Brenda Gregory).

Mandible

The mandible supports the teeth of the lower jaw. Two separate bones meeting at the rostral midline (symphysis) create the mandible. The mandibular symphysis is a fibrous joint. Unlike in humans, it is rare for this juncture to fuse completely in dogs and cats. Cats tend to have a very "loose" mandibular symphysis. The ends of the mandibles meet the temporal bone to form the temporomandibular joint or TMJ. It is a hinge joint. Muscles of mastication, originating along the cranium, insert into the body of the mandible near the TMJ. They provide the ability to open and close the mouth, eat, chew, and bite. In rare cases, the TMJ can luxate, preventing the animal from closing its mouth.

Incisive

The incisive bone is the rostral section of the maxilla. It supports the upper incisor teeth. Defects in the formation of this bone can cause a cleft palate.

Maxilla

Along with supporting the remainder, the upper canines, premolars, and molars, the maxilla also includes the palatine bones, creating the hard palate. The maxilla separates the oral cavity from the nasal cavity.

Muscles

Muscles of the skull allow movement, facial expression, chewing, eating, and biting. While these are not the sleek muscles of the limbs, the strong muscles of the face are designed to rip and tear food. They also create an extreme ability to bite. In humans, the biting force is 250–300 pounds per square inch (psi) with the ability to create a sudden snapping force of 25,000–30,000 psi. Contrast this to the canine with a normal range of 300–800 psi and the potential for 30,000–80,000 psi when provoked.

Nerves

The trigeminal nerve (cranial nerve V) begins at the brain stem and divides into three branches: ophthalmic, maxillary, and mandibular. The trigeminal nerve and its subsidiary branches provide sensory and motor function. To keep within the context of this chapter, we will only discuss the branches related to dentistry.

The maxillary nerve provides sensation to the lower eyelids, nasal mucosa, maxillary teeth, upper lip, and the nose. Branching from the maxillary nerve, the minor and major palatine nerves provide sensation to the soft and hard palates as well as giving rise to taste fibers. The infraorbital nerve branches into the three alveolar branches that enter the alveolar canal and each tooth root. The caudal superior, middle superior, and rostral superior alveolar nerves supply the maxillary molars, premolars, and canines/incisors, respectively.

The mandibular nerve provides motor function to the mouth by innervating muscles of biting and eating. The mandibular nerve and its many branches provide sensation to the cheeks, tongue, mandibular teeth, lower lip, and the skin of the head. The mandibular nerve branches into the masticator nerve, which aids in opening the mouth; the related masseteric and deep temporal nerves, which allow closing of the mouth; the lateral and medial pterygoid nerves, which aid in raising the mandible while eating; the buccal nerve, which provides sensation to the skin and mucosa of the cheek; the inferior alveolar nerve, which supplies sensation to all the mandibular teeth and exits the mandible through its mental nerve branches and foramina; the mental nerves, which provide sensation to the lower lip and rostral intermandibular region; and the lingual nerve, which creates tongue sensations of touch, pain, temperature, and taste.

Vascular System

Arteries

The external carotid artery and its branches supply blood flow to the oral cavity. The palatine branch runs ventrally in the lateral wall of the pharynx and provides blood supply to the palatine glands, mucosa, and muscles. Pharyngeal arteries serve the mucosa and muscle of the pharynx. The largest branch of the external carotid artery is the lingual. Running from the tip to the base of the tongue, it further bifurcates into the hyoid and tonsillar branches. The facial artery supplies blood flow to the mandibular and sublingual salivary glands and facial muscles and gives rise to the sublingual artery. Running parallel to the mandible, it supplies the rostral mandible and lower incisor teeth. The superficial temporal artery and its many branches bring blood to the parotid salivary gland, zygomatic arch, and temporal muscle. The maxillary artery divides into the mandibular and pterygopalatine branches. The mandibular portion supplies the TMJ and the roots of the mandibular teeth. It terminates at the mental arteries in the rostral mandible. The pterygopalatine portion gives rise to many branches. They provide blood flow to the eye, nose, sinuses, and facial muscles. The alveolar arteries, terminal branches of the maxillary artery, serve all the maxillary teeth.

Veins

Terminating in the external jugular vein, the arteries' corresponding veins drain blood from the head. These include the lingual-facial, facial, mandibular, temporal, and maxillary veins.

Lymphatic System

The following lymph nodes of the head are of importance in dentistry:

- The parotid lymph nodes lie at the level of the TMJ and are rostral to the parotid salivary gland
- Mandibular lymph nodes are rostroventral to the mandibular salivary glands
- Retropharyngeal lymph nodes are deep and caudal to the mandibular salivary gland and dorsolateral and caudal to the pharynx

Dental conditions, gingivitis, and periodontal disease can manifest themselves with enlargement of the adjacent lymph nodes.

Eye

Although the eye is not an organ involved with oral anatomy, the close approximation between the two systems mean that it should be considered. Infected and

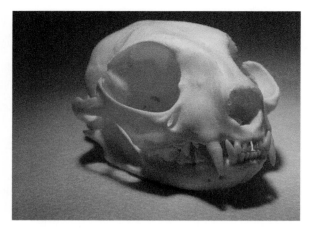

Figure 1.10   Cat skull showing the minimal distance between the infraorbital foramen and the eye socket.

abscessed maxillary premolars or molars may present as suborbital swelling. There is little distance between the orbit and the infraorbital foramen, especially in the cat, and care should be taken when administering regional nerve block in this area to avoid puncture of the eye (Fig. 1.10).

Larynx and Pharynx

The oral cavity and oral portion of the respiratory system coincide during their formation. The larynx is the oral opening to the trachea and lungs. The epiglottis closes to prevent food from entering the trachea. The pharynx opens into the esophagus to provide passage of food. The tonsils are located within the pharyngeal opening. Tonsils are modified lymph tissue and changes in them can be indicative of disease.

Odontogenesis[5]

Odontogenesis is the development of teeth (odont = tooth, genesis = origin). The development of the gastrointestinal (GI) tract, including the oral cavity and teeth, is a complex series of events. In the embryo, the GI tract begins as an endodermic tube. Within a short period, this structure folds in on itself to form three distinct sections: foregut, midgut, and hindgut. The foregut gives rise to the pharynx, esophagus, stomach, duodenum, respiratory tract, liver, gallbladder, and pancreas. The midgut becomes the jejunum, ileum, cecum, appendix, ascending colon, and part of the transverse colon. The hindgut forms the rest of the transverse colon, rectum, and anal canal. The oral cavity develops from the pharyngeal end of the foregut as the oral plate. From this, the maxilla, mandible, and their associated structures form.

Tooth Formation[6]

Teeth form from the gathering of mesenchymal cells from the ectoderm along the epithelium of the mandible and maxilla at specific sites.[7] A variety of growth factors

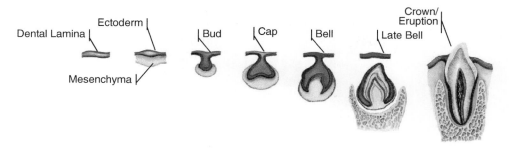

Figure 1.11 Tooth development (Illustration by Brenda Gregory).

interact with this follicle to form the tooth bud. Additional growth factors create the enamel knot and the cap stage of development when the tooth cells begin to align. During the cap stage, nerves and blood vessels begin to develop and enter the developing dentin, eventually becoming the pulp of the tooth. The bell stage then follows and begins the differentiation into the tooth components of dentin and enamel. In the final, crown stage, enamel forms with the mineralization of odontoblasts. Ameloblasts aid in the creation of enamel toward the outer surface of the developing tooth. Odontoblasts move toward the center of the tooth creating dentin. (Secondary dentin continues to form in permanent teeth throughout life, causing a gradual narrowing of the pulp chamber.) Cementoblasts form the cementum in the very late stages of tooth development (Fig. 1.11).

Eruption[8]

Many theories exist on the mechanism of tooth eruption. The three current theories are as follows.

- **Root formation:** As the tooth root develops, it elongates the tooth, pushing it through the gingival tissues; however, rootless teeth develop.
- **Alveolar bone remodeling:** Bone formation at the apex of the tooth and resorption of bone at the coronal end of the tooth follicle interact to create penetration of the mucosa.
- **Periodontal ligament:** Periodontal ligament formation and renewal are involved in the continuous growth of teeth in some species (e.g., rodents and rabbits); however, this has not been proven in species of animals with only two sets of teeth.

If there is no path for the eruption of a tooth, it may become impacted or embedded. An impacted tooth is one prevented by bone from erupting. Soft tissue inhibits an embedded tooth's eruption. If there is a disruption of a tooth bud during development, it may grow in an abnormal location or create a dentigerous cyst (Fig. 1.12).

Primary teeth

Dogs and cats are diphyodont, with two sets of teeth during their lifetime. As the permanent teeth erupt, the roots of the primary (deciduous) teeth are absorbed, so they become loose and eventually fall out. Other species, such as most rodents and

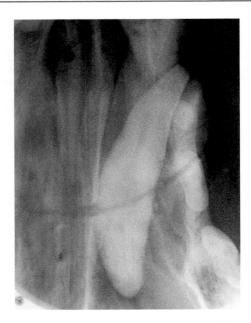

Figure 1.12   Radiograph of the permanent upper right canine tooth of a dog bitten in the face as a puppy. Note the development of the tooth within the nasal sinus.

Table 1.1   Primary tooth eruption schedule

Tooth type	Canine (week of eruption)	Feline (week of eruption)
Incisors	3–4	2–3
Canines	3	3–4
Premolars	4–12	3–6
Molars	None	None

lagomorphs, have open-rooted teeth that continue to grow throughout their life. Many types of snakes and sharks are polyphyodont and continuously replace teeth as they exfoliate. Table 1.1 shows the tooth eruption schedule for primary teeth of dogs and cats.

Permanent teeth

Primary and permanent teeth do not fall out and erupt at the same rate. A mixed dentition is often present. Normally, as the permanent tooth emerges, the primary tooth is lost. If this does not occur, the primary tooth is retained. Two teeth should not occupy the same space at the same time. Retained primary teeth can lead to rotation and malocclusion of the permanent teeth. The close interdigitation of the primary and permanent tooth prevents thorough cleaning, causing food and debris to accumulate. This may lead to periodontal disease. Abnormal interdigitation

Table 1.2   Permanent tooth eruption schedule

Tooth type	Canine (month of eruption)	Feline (month of eruption)
Incisors	3–5	3–4
Canines	4–6	4–5
Premolars	4–6	4–6
Molars	5–7	4–5

may cause long-term damage to the developing permanent tooth and potential tooth loss.

The timing of tooth eruption varies with sex, breed, overall health and well-being, body size, and season of birth. Teeth of females, larger breeds, summer-born, and healthy animals erupt earlier than their counterparts. Table 1.2 shows the permanent tooth eruption schedule for dogs and cats.

Anatomy of the Tooth

Every tooth, no matter its form or function, contains the same elements. Multirooted teeth have additional structures but internally are equivalent to single-rooted teeth. The tooth structures are crown, enamel, cementum, dentin, pulp, root, and periodontal ligament (Fig. 1.13).

Crown

The crown is the most visible portion of the tooth and is primarily made of enamel. The tip of a crown is the cusp. It meets the tooth root at the cementoenamel junction (CEJ), also known as the neck or cervical line. Crowns are subject to wear, fractures, and discolorations. Wear occurs from excessive chewing on rocks, cages, tennis balls, sticks, and so on. Fractures are the result of trauma. Discoloration can be the result of tetracycline or doxycycline administration during tooth formation, causing the teeth to turn yellow. Trauma may also cause discoloration, resulting from injury to the internal tooth structures. In a vital tooth, the injured tooth is pink to red from hemorrhage within the pulp. If left untreated, the tooth may "die" or become non-vital. The crown will then become purple, gray, or black.

Enamel

Enamel covers the crown of the tooth. The strongest surface in the body, enamel is composed primarily of mineral with a small quantity of water and organic matter. It is shiny and varies in color from white to ivory. Canine teeth are often more bright white than human teeth. The mineral content creates the strength of the enamel but

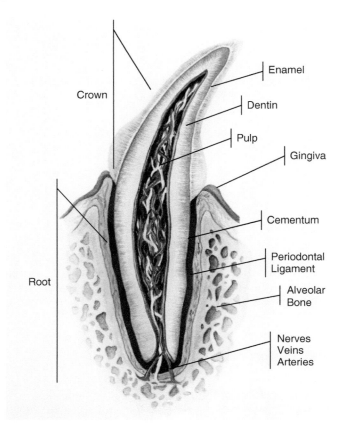

Figure 1.13 Anatomy of a tooth (Illustration by Brenda Gregory).

also makes it brittle. Enamel chip fractures are a common finding when animals chew on hard surfaces such as rocks and bones. Due to the absence of a blood supply, enamel cannot heal itself when injured. In the adult dog, enamel is approximately 1 mm in depth. In young animals, enamel easily fractures because it is fragile with a large underlying pulp chamber. See Dentin.

Cementum

Cementum is mineralized connective tissue covering the root of the tooth. It begins at the CEJ and continues apically. The CEJ or "neck" of the tooth is the location where the enamel and cementum meet. Unlike shiny enamel, cementum is dull and often pitted. The lower mineral content of cementum makes it softer than enamel, dentin, and bone. Collagen fibers of the periodontal ligament penetrate cementum to aid in retention of the root in the alveolar bone.

Dentin

The majority of a tooth is made of dentin, which is 70% inorganic material with the remainder being collagen fibers and water. Dentin is porous and yellowish in color.

Made up of odontoblasts (odonto = tooth, blast = germ or embryo), the dentin continues to fill in the pulp cavity of a vital tooth. This continual laying down of odontoblasts causes the pulp cavity/root canal to narrow with age. There are three primary types of dentin. Primary dentin forms prior to a tooth's eruption. Secondary dentin develops after eruption and through life. Trauma to the tooth causes the formation of tertiary dentin. This reparative material may be brown or a darker yellow than the surrounding tooth structure.

Pulp

The pulp is the most vital portion of a tooth. Veins, arteries, lymphatic vessels, nerves, odontoblasts, and other cellular structures make up the pulp or endodontic (endo = within, dontic = tooth) system. The pulp chamber joins the periodontal ligament at the apex of the tooth. The coronal or crown section and the root section (root canal) divide the tooth into two areas. The structures of the pulp provide nourishment, sensation, and defense. The veins and arteries keep the tooth alive. The nerves react to trauma by transmitting pain sensation. Odontoblasts from the pulp form dentin. As noted earlier, the pulp chamber continues to narrow throughout life, from the continuous deposition of odontoblasts. Damage to a tooth early in life may cause pulp inflammation or death, stopping odontoblast production and resulting in a large pulp chamber.

A variety of insults cause tooth death and loss by injuring the pulp. Crowns with no gross sign of trauma may be discolored, indicating internal trauma to the pulp. In an intact tooth, the pulp chamber is a closed space. Swelling within the pulp chamber often leads to pulpal necrosis from internal pressure applied to the arteries, cutting off blood supply to the tooth. If left untreated, impact trauma that creates a tooth fracture with an open pulp chamber often leads to tooth death. Aggressive and improper use of dental power tools – scalers, polishers, and drills – may cause excessive heat buildup within the pulp chamber, resulting in inflammation. Bacteria from untreated periodontal disease or bacteremia can ascend into the pulp chamber causing pulpitis and necrosis. Without treatment, bacterial pulpitis may spread apically (toward the apex or root), creating an abscess and alveolar bone loss.

Roots

Tooth roots contain the living tissues of the tooth. Composed mostly of dentin and covered with cementum, roots anchor the tooth with the attached periodontal ligament. The tip of the root is the apex. Dog and cat teeth have an apical delta composed of several openings leading into the pulp chamber or root canal. Human teeth have a single opening. The importance of the apical delta becomes evident during endodontic (root canal) therapy.

In dogs, the incisors, canines, first premolars, and the third mandibular molars are all single rooted. The only three-rooted teeth in dogs are the maxillary fourth premolars and first and second molars. All other teeth have two roots. In cats, the incisors, canines, maxillary second premolars, and molars have one root. The rest of the teeth are double-rooted except the fourth maxillary premolar – the only three-rooted tooth in the cat mouth (Table 1.3). The space between roots in a multirooted tooth is the furcation. It is the area where the roots bifurcate or divide.

Table 1.3 Tooth root numbers

Tooth	Canine		Feline	
	Maxilla	Mandible	Maxilla	Mandible
Incisors – all	1	1	1	1
Canines – all	1	1	1	1
First premolar	1	1	Absent	Absent
Second premolar	2	2	1	Absent
Third premolar	2	2	2	2
Fourth premolar	3	2	3	2
First molar	3	2	1	2
Second molar	3	2	Absent	Absent
Third molar	Absent	1	Absent	Absent

Periodontal Ligament

The periodontal ligament attaches the cementum of the tooth to the alveolar bone and the cementum of adjoining teeth. Collagen fibers are its primary component, but it also contains blood vessels, nerves, and elastic fibers. The strong fibers of the periodontal ligament counteract forces put onto teeth from chewing, trauma, and extraction. The elasticity of the ligament allows the tooth to move slightly during normal activity. Strong forces from either trauma or extraction are required to dislodge a tooth. Unlike the nerves within the pulp cavity, the nerves of the periodontal ligament contribute to the sensations of pressure, heat, and cold.

Inflammation of the gingiva (gingivitis) is an ascending condition leading to periodontal disease – the number one most common condition in dogs and cats. Periodontitis (inflammation of the periodontium) destroys the periodontal ligament, gingiva, bone, and eventually results in tooth loss. It is a treatable condition if managed in its early stages (see web content: Video 1.1W Dental anatomy).

Directional Terminology[9]

The mouth has its own terminology related to the location of the tooth, the direction in the mouth, and position related to the tongue and cheeks. Learning this terminology will aid the veterinary technician in performing an oral exam and assisting the veterinarian. The following terms relate to the tooth surface (see Fig. 1.14) and (see web content: Video 1.2W Directional terminology):

- **Mesial:** Toward the midline of the face
- **Distal:** Away from the midline of the face

(a)

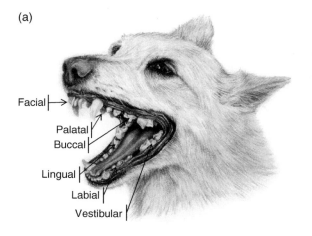

Facial

Palatal

Buccal

Lingual

Labial

Vestibular

(b)

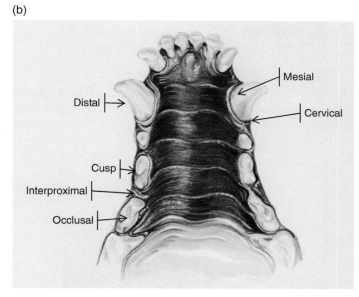

Distal

Mesial

Cervical

Cusp

Interproximal

Occlusal

Figure 1.14 Directional terminology (Illustration by Brenda Gregory).

- **Vestibular:** Toward the vestibule or lips (interchangeable with labial or buccal)
- **Labial:** Toward the lips, used for the incisors and canines
- **Buccal:** Toward the cheeks, used for premolars and molars
- **Facial:** Surfaces of rostral teeth visible from the front
- **Lingual:** Toward the tongue, used in the mandible
- **Palatal:** Toward the palate, used in the maxilla
- **Coronal:** Toward the crown of the tooth
- **Apical:** Toward the root of the tooth
- **Contact, proximal, or occlusal:** Toward adjoining teeth in the same jaw
- **Interproximal:** Between two teeth
- **Cusp:** Point of the tooth
- **Cervical or neck:** Area of the tooth where crown and root meet

Abbreviations

Abbreviations aid dental charting and record keeping. The two primary forms of abbreviation for tooth identification in veterinary dentistry are the proper identification sequence and the Triadan system. Abbreviations for oral pathology are discussed in Chapter 5. The American Veterinary Dental College (AVDC) continuously updates the abbreviations.

Proper identification sequence

This version of tooth identification involves using dentition (permanent or primary – indicated with lower case "d" for deciduous), arch (maxilla/mandible, often upper/lower), quadrant (left or right), and tooth (using tooth formula abbreviations: I, C, PM, and M). For example, for the proper identification of the permanent mandibular left first molar using subscripts and superscripts to identify the arch and quadrant, the shorthand is $_1M$. The primary (deciduous) maxillary right third incisor is indicated as dI^3.

Triadan system

Adopted by the AVDC, the Triadan system identifies each tooth with a three-digit number. The first number indicates the quadrant of the tooth's location and its dentition (primary or permanent): maxillary right = 1 (5 for primary), maxillary left = 2 (6), mandibular left = 3 (7), and mandibular right = 4 (8). Based on the full dentition of a pig, second and third numbers follow sequentially, with incisors being

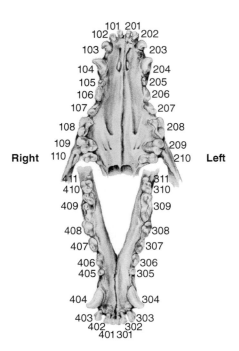

Figure 1.15 Canine Triadan tooth numbering system (Illustration by Brenda Gregory).

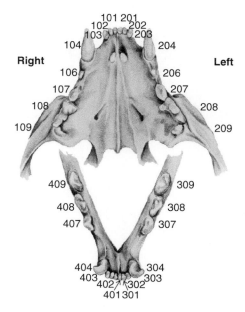

Figure 1.16 Feline Triadan tooth numbering system (Illustration by Brenda Gregory).

numbers 01, 02, and 03, canines = 04, premolars = 05, 06, 07, and 08, and molars = 09, 10, 11. Adult cats normally are missing the maxillary first premolar and mandibular first and second premolars. The numbering system remains intact by skipping these missing teeth. An easy device for implementing the Triadan system is the canine teeth are always number 4, and the fourth premolars are always number 8. Using the above examples, the permanent mandibular left first molar is tooth 309. The primary (deciduous) maxillary right third incisor is tooth number 503. A cat's permanent right mandibular fourth premolar, even though it is the second premolar found in the mouth, is tooth number 408. Remember, cats normally are missing teeth 405 and 406 (Figs. 1.15 and 1.16 and see web content: Video 1.3W Tooth numbering).

See Appendices 2 and 3 for sample canine and feline dental charts.

References

1. Evans, HE. 1993. *Miller's Anatomy of the Dog*, 3rd edn. Philadelphia, PA: Saunders.
2. Wiggs, RB, Lobprise, HB. 1997. *Veterinary Dentistry Principles and Practice.* Philadelphia, PA: Lippincott-Raven.
3. Gioso, MA, Carvalho, VGG, Holmstrom, SE (editors). 2005. *Oral Anatomy of the Dog and Cat, Veterinary Clinics of North America, Small Animal Practice-Dentistry*. Philadelphia, PA: Saunders.
4. Budras, KD, McCarthy, PH, Horowitz, A, Berg, R. 2006. *Anatomy of the Dog*, 5th edn. Hanover: Schlütersche.
5. Gilbert, SF. 2006. *Tooth Development – Developmental Biology*, 8th edn online. Sunderland, MA: Sinauer Associates.

6. Harvey, CE, Emily, PP. 1993. *Small Animal Dentistry*. St. Louis, MO: Mosby.
7. Theslaff, I. 2003. Epithelial-mesenchymal signaling regulating tooth morphogenesis. *Journal of Cell Science* 116:1647–1648.
8. Johnson, C. 2001. *Mechanisms of tooth eruption*. University of Illinois at Chicago Courses online: Oral Sciences.
9. Holmstrom, SE. 2000. *Veterinary Dentistry for the Technician and Office Staff*. Philadelphia, PA: Saunders.

The Examination Room and the Dental Patient

2

Mary Berg, BS, RLATG, RVT, VTS (Dentistry)

Learning Objectives

- Conduct an effective client interview
- Gather an accurate history
- Perform an oral examination on the conscious patient
- Prepare and present a treatment estimate to the client
- Convey the importance of the recommended dental procedure to the client

Small Animal Dental Procedures for Veterinary Technicians and Nurses, Second Edition.
Edited by Jeanne R. Perrone.
© 2021 John Wiley & Sons, Inc. Published 2021 by John Wiley & Sons, Inc.

Introduction

The veterinarian is the only one who can make a diagnosis of disease, but the veterinary technician/nurse and staff can assist the veterinarian by gathering an accurate history and recognizing pathology and bring it to the attention of the veterinarian. The veterinary technician/nurse plays a vital role in a successful dental practice. Each practice should have a veterinary technician/nurse whose main emphasis is in dentistry.[1] This veterinary technician/nurse's responsibilities include client education, communication, and therapeutic skills, as well as educating the remainder of the staff. The dental veterinary technician/nurse is responsible for gathering an accurate history and performing an oral examination on the pet prior to the doctor's examination. By doing so, they are able to give the veterinarian an accurate evaluation of the pet. Veterinary technician/nurses should develop a good understanding of all aspects of veterinary dentistry in order to field questions that clients may ask. In a successful dental practice, all members of the veterinary staff play an important role in caring for the patient.[1]

The Client Interview

Veterinarians need to use a combination of knowledge and observation in dentistry, comparing abnormal findings with known normals to determine the best course of treatment. Part of gathering the information needed to develop that treatment plan is gathering an accurate history on the patient by interviewing the client. This history should be gathered by the veterinary technician/nurse. This allows the doctor to enter the exam room with an understanding of the oral condition of the pet.

Some clients are astute owners and are able to recognize that there is a problem with their pet's oral cavity; however, many seem to be unaware that their pet even has teeth![1,2] When a client presents a pet they suspect has a problem with the oral cavity, it is necessary to interview the client to gather the needed information as well as perform an oral exam of the pet. As veterinary professionals we have to rely on the pet owner's description of the symptoms.[2] These symptoms may commonly include malodor, and more rarely excessive salivation, inappetance, swelling, difficulty swallowing, or indications of oral pain or discomfort.[2] This information, along with the complete history including past oral examinations and treatments, diet, chewing habits, and home care, are all pieces of the puzzle that must be put together.[2]

Sometimes the owner is not even aware that there is a problem with their pet's mouth. Oftentimes, the dental problems are discovered during the oral portion of the annual examination. They may have noticed a change but did not think it was relevant or important. This is the perfect time to educate the client on oral disease and its importance to the animal's overall health.

The past history of the patient is valuable information that can aid the veterinary staff in determining the treatment plan.[1] Having a complete history of past oral examinations and treatments helps the veterinarian understand the present oral condition and predict the outcome of a procedure. A 10-year-old toy breed dog that has not had any previous oral examinations and/or treatments is likely to have severe oral disease, while a similar patient that has had annual dental cleanings may only have mild disease.

Just as a veterinary technician/nurse interviews the client regarding lifestyle to assist the veterinarian in determining the appropriate vaccine protocol, the veterinary technician/nurse should ask many questions when interviewing the client about the pet's oral health. Encourage the client to volunteer information if possible, but some questions need to be asked. A nonleading question is the best way to gather information.

If a client is not aware of any problems with their pet's oral cavity, questions that should be asked are as follows:

- Has Ricky had any previous dental work? Let the owner volunteer information for you. Yes, Ricky did have two teeth extracted at my previous veterinarian. At this point you can ask more pointed questions regarding the cause for the extractions, when the procedure was performed, and so on.
- Is Jaxx a heavy chewer? He used to be but you know lately he has had no interest in his toys or bones.
- What is Poppy's favorite chew toy? Some pets are very orally fixated, while others may not be chewers. Some toys, such as tennis balls, ice, cow hooves, pig ears, and hard nylon bones, can cause serious trauma in the mouth.[1] Clients may not realize the harm that could come from what they thought was a great toy. Use this opportunity to educate your clients about possible harm.

If the client is aware of a problem, ask them when they first noticed a problem. Oral disease can develop slowly and the owner may not be aware of the problem. Many owners think that bad breath is normal in their pet and are not aware that periodontal disease may be the culprit.[3] Nevertheless, malodor does not always mean periodontal disease; other forms of dental disease and/or gastrointestinal disease may also be the cause.[3]

The following questions should be asked in situations where the owner is concerned about a problem:

- Has your pet had any problems eating? Do they tend to drop food or chew on one side of the mouth? Have they stopped eating altogether or will only eat soft food?
- Does your pet seem to salivate excessively?
- Does your pet appear to have problems drinking or swallowing?
- Has there been a change in your pet's habits or behavior?
- Does your pet rub its face on the carpet or paw at their face? Face rubbing can be a sign of oral pain or inflammation.

In traumatic cases, such as a fractured, avulsed, or luxated tooth, it is vital to know when the injury happened if there is to be a chance of saving the tooth.

The Oral Examination: Conscious Patient

The general health exam is performed by the veterinarian. During the examination the entire animal should be examined from nose to tail. A thorough exam should include the eyes, ears, skin, heart, lung, abdomen, and check for internal parasites. If anesthesia is planned, it is highly recommended to perform blood and urine analysis. Preanesthetic testing is discussed in more detail in Chapter 4.

The oral examination is done on both the conscious and the anesthetized patient. The conscious exam is limited to olfactory, visual, and tactile examination. A primary indication of oral disease is malodor.[1,3] A normal, healthy breath will have a sweaty, salty odor but is not unpleasant.[3] Periodontal disease is usually accompanied by a strong, unpleasant odor comparable to necrosis and infection.[3]

Evaluate the symmetry of the head. Do both sides appear to be uniform or does one side look different?[2] Is there swelling in any area of the head? If swelling appears below the eye, look for a fractured maxillary fourth premolar. Do the jaws appear symmetrical? If one side of the jaw is swollen or not symmetrical, rule out mandibular or tooth fractures, or oral masses.

Feel the head. Palpate the bones of the head including the zygomatic arch and mandibles. Feel for the presence of abnormalities. Evaluate the lymph nodes, including the sublingual and submandibular nodes. Inflammation in the oral cavity can contribute to swelling of these nodes. The temporomandibular joint should also be palpated for indications of pain or discomfort.

A cursory oral exam should be performed prior to anesthesia if possible. During this exam, check for occlusion, tooth fractures, gingival recession and inflammation, and missing, supernumerary, or loose teeth. If your patient is cooperative, show the client the areas of concern (Fig. 2.1).

Malocclusion is the improper alignment of the teeth. It is discussed fully in Chapter 7 but it is important to evaluate this prior to anesthesia and intubation. It is important to look at all of the teeth to evaluate occlusion, not just the incisors. Begin by ensuring that the incisors meet in a healthy and comfortable bite. The maxillary incisors are rostral to the mandibular incisors. The mandibular canine teeth should fit into the diastema between the maxillary third incisor and the maxillary canine. The premolars should have a pinking shears appearance, with the cusps of the premolars opposing the interdental spaces of the opposing arcade. The maxillary first premolar should be the most rostral. The maxillary fourth premolar should occlude

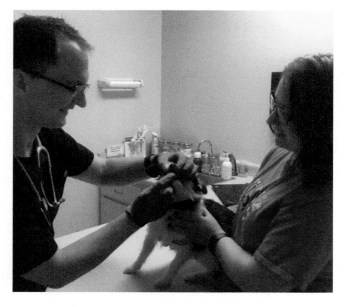

Figure 2.1   The veterinary technician evaluates the occlusion and oral condition of the pet in the exam room. This is a perfect time to educate your client about the oral health status of their pet.

along the buccal surface of the mandibular first molar. There are certain breeds in which malocclusion would be considered a normal bite for the breed. For example, boxers have an underbite or mandibular mesioclusion. Use the American Kennel Club breed standards as a reference for the type of bites that are acceptable in each breed. This will be reviewed in the "Malocclusion" section in Chapter 7.

Count the teeth to determine if there are supernumerary teeth present or if teeth are missing. This task can be difficult as not every patient is willing to allow a good look, especially if they are head shy or a young puppy. Dental formulae are listed in Chapter 1.

Each tooth should be evaluated for fractures, mobility, and the amount of plaque and calculus present.

Although it is most important to evaluate the gingiva under general anesthesia when the gingival index and pocket depth can be evaluated, it is useful to observe the gingiva preanathesia to determine a preliminary degree of periodontal inflammation. Healthy gingiva is pink with defined margins, while inflammation is indicated by red, swollen gums. Gingival recession or hyperplasia are key elements of periodontal disease and should be noted.

A complete examination can only be completed under general anesthesia and will be covered in Chapter 5; however, the exam on the conscious patient can yield vital information that can help create the treatment plan for the patient and estimate for the client.

Communicating with Clients

Clients rely on the veterinary team to provide them with clear and accurate information. Unfortunately, sometimes the team may have difficulty in conveying a message to the pet owner. Terms may be used that the client does not understand or slang is used that may not convey the importance of the message. Communicating with clients about dental procedures is no different. It is important to use terms that help the pet owners grasp the importance of dentistry. Here are a few terms that should be avoided and terms that can substituted to gain compliance with medical needs.

- A **"dental"**: This is sometimes loosely used as a slang term that pet owners often do not fully understand and may think is only a tooth brushing. It can be replaced with professional dental cleaning, COHAT (comprehensive oral health assessment and treatment), OAT (oral assessment and treatment), ATP (assessment and treatment plan), or periodontal therapy. These terms are more descriptive of the actual procedure and let the pet owner know that this is a medically needed treatment.
- **Prophy:** Unfortunately most dental procedures are not prophylactic procedures but treatment of oral disease that is already present. It is to be hoped that someday we will truly be performing prophies on the majority of our patients.
- **Periodontal disease:** Clients may not truly understand this term unless they have it themselves. Use the terms "infection" and "pain" instead. Clients understand infection and pain. Although periodontal disease begins as an inflammatory response to the bacteria in plaque, it develops into an infection of the tissues surrounding the teeth and can be painful to our pets.
- **Recommend:** Replace recommend with need. Do not say "The doctor recommends a professional dental cleaning." A recommendation is just a suggestion.

Say instead "Your pet *needs* a professional dental cleaning." Replace *should* with *need* and *could* with *must*. This helps to tell the owner this is important and needs to be taken care of soon. If an owner hears "The pet needs to have a professional dental cleaning and it must be scheduled soon to prevent the infection from getting worse and risking tooth loss and systemic health problems" they are more likely to schedule the procedure instead of waiting.

The Dental Estimate (Treatment Plan)

The best veterinarians will not be able to practice their dental skills if the owner does not give permission. The veterinary technician/nurse's role in obtaining this permission includes creating an accurate treatment plan for the procedure and presenting the plan to the client. The client needs to understand the pathology and the need for therapy. The veterinary technician/nurse plays a vital role in providing this education to the client.

The treatment plan should be itemized and as accurate as possible. The veterinary technician/nurse should go through it with the client, explaining the need for and value of each item.

For example:

- Preanesthetic blood work can sometimes find systemic problems that have a bearing on the anesthesia protocol and inform the patient's anesthetic risk (see Chapter 4).
- Dental radiographs are necessary to determine if there is pathology that is not visible on the crown.

Explaining the treatment plan line by line helps the client understand the need for and importance of the treatment. Use photographs, models, videos, and charts to let the clients see the pathology. Clients may see and understand the pathology more easily in pictures than in the oral cavity of their pet (Figs. 2.2 and 2.3).

It is good practice to provide a treatment plan or estimate to the client prior to each procedure. This practice prevents distress over unexpected expenses and helps the client understand that the procedure is important to their pet's health. Providing an estimate in advance can also help the client make arrangements for payments.

An exact treatment plan cannot be determined in the exam room on a conscious patient, but a close "estimate" can be created from the oral exam. Explain that the treatment plan is only an estimate and that a more accurate plan can be prepared once the animal is under anesthesia and the final oral exam and dental radiographs have been performed. Creating an estimate higher than anticipated can have a twofold benefit. First, it allows for an allowance if the periodontal disease is more advanced than thought on the initial exam. Second, the client can be pleasantly surprised to have a lower cost for the procedure. If the client would like a more precise estimate prior to the procedure, prepare a "worst-case scenario" and explain this to the client.

An understanding of the owner's commitment and ability to perform home care will help develop your treatment plan.[1] If you have an understanding of your client's degree of commitment, your veterinarian may plan to perform periodontal surgery to save teeth or decide to extract the teeth in the best interest of the pet.

See Appendices 4 and 5 for dental procedure estimate and release form.

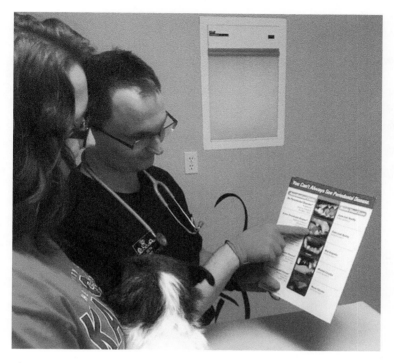

Figure 2.2   The veterinary technician uses diagrams to illustrate the link between oral health and systemic health.

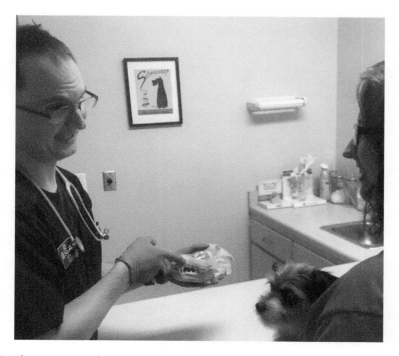

Figure 2.3   The veterinary technician uses a skull as an aid to explain the pet's oral health to the client.

CHAPTER 2

References

1. Bellows, J. 1999. *The Practice of Veterinary Dentistry: A Team Effort.* Ames, IA: Iowa State Press.
2. Lobprise, HB, Wiggs, RB. 2000. *The Veterinarian's Companion for Common Dental Procedures.* Lakewood, CO: AAHA Press.
3. Lobprise, HB, Dodd, JR. 2019. *Wigg's Veterinary Dentistry Principles and Practice*, 2nd edn. Hoboken, NJ: Wiley Blackwell.

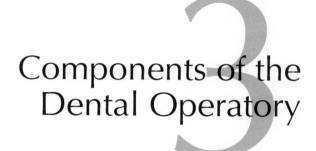

Components of the Dental Operatory

Benita Altier, LVT, VTS (Dentistry)

Learning Objectives

- Identify all equipment and infrastructure needed in the veterinary dental operatory
- Recognize the importance of all components and understand the basic principles of setting up equipment for use
- Gain an understanding of how to organize the dental operatory for ergonomic safety and efficiency of the dental team
- Become familiar with various dental delivery units and their specific uses
- Understand the use of air compression versus motor-driven systems and the benefits and limitations of each type
- Recognize ways that we can use ergonomic principles to create operator comfort when utilizing the dental delivery unit
- Become familiar with the different types of handpieces that are used for veterinary dentistry
- Learn techniques to maintain the instruments' usefulness by proper daily care of the equipment
- Recognize the different types of ultrasonic scalers available as well as how they operate and function optimally
- Gain an understanding of how the dental table and chairs can affect the way that we perform procedures, efficiency, and patient and operator comfort
- Use a neutral seated posture to maintain the normal curvature of the spine and avoid musculoskeletal injuries and disorders
- Know what types of hazards are present in the dental operatory
- Recognize and learn how to use personal protective equipment during dental procedures

Small Animal Dental Procedures for Veterinary Technicians and Nurses, Second Edition.
Edited by Jeanne R. Perrone.
© 2021 John Wiley & Sons, Inc. Published 2021 by John Wiley & Sons, Inc.

Components of the Dental Operatory: The Big Picture

The dental operatory should provide the following:

- Sufficient dedicated space to practice dentistry, outside of any high-traffic areas and away from sterile surgical rooms
- An adjustable-height or stationary table(s) sufficient in size for larger dogs
- Surgical lighting and personal focal lighting and magnification
- A dental radiology unit, wall or floor mounted, with space for a laptop computer or a similar wall-mounted monitor to view and control radiology software
- A dental delivery system consisting of an onboard or off-site air compressor, high- and low-speed handpieces, air–water syringe, as well as an ultrasonic scaler. Optional handpieces could include an additional high-speed handpiece, suction, and light-emitting diode (LED) light sources
- Anesthesia machine – wall-, cabinet-, or floor-mounted model with adequate scavenging systems
- Active warming device to prevent patient hypothermia
- Intravenous fluid pump mounted on wall or cabinet
- Storage for all dentistry-related supplies and items
- Tray for dental instrumentation during the procedure
- Ergonomic seating for the operator(s)
- Anesthetic monitoring machine or devices

Operatory Functionality

The dental operatory should provide plenty of unobstructed room for a dedicated team member to efficiently perform anesthetic monitoring.

Use of an active warming system and careful temperature monitoring by the dedicated team member will ensure that the patient remains normothermic throughout the procedure. Placement for these units should be planned carefully within the dental space, to allow for easy access when using the device.

The equipment in the dental operatory should be oriented and organized in a way that enables the operator to access the dental delivery unit and handpieces, hand instruments, and patient without twisting, extensive reaching, or leaving a seated position.

Ergonomically correct seating that is suitable for each person should be available. The best chairs encourage a neutral spinal posture.

All equipment should be well maintained and safety checks carried out before patient induction to ensure the equipment is functioning correctly.

Lighting should be focal to the operatory field and be of significant strength to illuminate the area. The operator's vision should be magnified approximately 2.5 times to provide adequate visualization of the oral structures.

Preparing the Dental Operatory for Procedures

Each component in the dental operatory should be inspected for cleanliness, disinfection or sterility, and function before use at the beginning of the day and in between each patient.

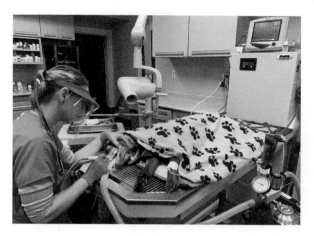

Figure 3.1   Dental operatory at Animal Hospital by the Sea, in Langley, Washington (Courtesy of Dr. Jean Dieden, DVM).

Dental radiology equipment should be powered on, ensuring the generator, sensor or phosphor plates, and scanner are ready, and the correct patient information entered into the software system (see Chapter 6 for more details).

The anesthetic machine, vaporizer, tubing, oxygen, scavenger, and all components should be carefully maintained, disinfected, and inspected before each patient. Similarly, the anesthetic monitoring equipment, patient warming device, and intravenous fluid pump should all be correctly set up and confirmed to be in working order.

The water supply to the dental delivery unit must be filled with mineral-free, distilled water and the unit should be plugged into an electricity supply, which is required to run the unit's air compressor as well as the ultrasonic scaler.[1-4] The low-speed handpiece should be equipped with a new disposable polishing angle, seated and locked into place using the locking mechanism on the handpiece.[1,2,4] The ultrasonic scaler's handpiece should be fitted with a sterilized scaler tip, appropriate for the level of calculus and area to be scaled.[2] The tips should be measured for working length on the particular unit's tip card before use.[1-4]

The table should be clean and covered with a thick towel to prevent loss of patient body heat through conduction into the table (Fig. 3.1).[2,5] The table height should be adjusted so the operator can sit comfortably around the end of the table while working. Towels or absorbent material can be placed under the patient's head after induction to absorb water spray from the ultrasonic scaler or high-speed handpiece. These should be changed as necessary to keep the patient dry and help prevent hypothermia.[2,5]

The dental instrumentation for periodontal cleaning and treatment should be opened sterilely and set aside on the procedure tray (Fig. 3.2).

Oral surgery packs and the high-speed handpiece should remain in sterile wrapping until the need for these items has been determined after dental radiographs and charting procedures are complete.

Dental Delivery Units

A dental delivery unit consists of several components, including a compressor and handpieces that are required to provide dental treatment to the veterinary patient. Each

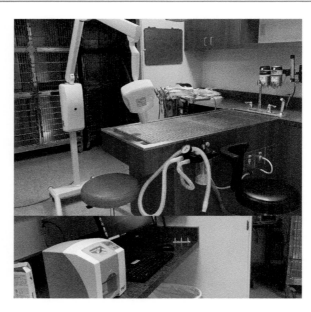

Figure 3.2   Dental operatory at Cheyenne West Animal Hospital, Las Vegas, Nevada (Courtesy of Dr. Brian Hewitt, DVM, DAVDC).

type of unit has its unique characteristics and maintenance procedures. The manual for the unit should always be consulted for specifics of use and maintenance.

Air- or Gas-Driven Units

An air-driven unit is composed of an electric motor-driven compressor which is either air or oil cooled (Fig. 3.3).[1,2,4] Air is pressurized in the tank to around 100 pounds per square inch (psi), then delivered at a lower pressure of 30–40 psi to high- and low-speed handpieces when the foot pedal is engaged.[1] Compressors that have oil-cooled motors require more maintenance than those with air-cooled motors.[1]

Alternatively, compressed nitrogen gas tanks can be used to drive the handpieces if a standard compressor is not available.[2] Nitrogen is a clean source of gas power for the handpieces; this gas power is an excellent option to help extend the life of the handpieces and reduce maintenance.[2]

A critical component of the dental unit is its ability to deliver water into the hand-pieces to flush away debris and to cool burs or tips that become heated due to friction, which could cause tissue or tooth damage or death.[1-4] Most dental delivery units use a bottle system to deliver distilled water into the handpieces; some have connections to attach a water source. An in-line filter attached to the tubing inside the water bottle will prevent contaminants from entering the water-lines and maintain a purer water supply. Some dental delivery units also have integrated ultrasonic scaling units, suction capabilities, and transillumination lighting and multiple stations for high-speed handpieces.[1]

Fiber optic lighting through an LED source can be built into the high-speed and ultrasonic scaler handpieces for complete visualization of the working area.

Air-driven handpieces can run at higher speeds than motor-driven scalers and polishers.[1,4]

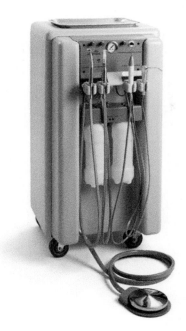

Figure 3.3   Midmark 1000™ dental delivery system with integrated piezoelectric scaler (Courtesy of the Midmark Corp).

Dental delivery units can stand alone in the dental operatory or may be integrated into dental tables or mounted on a wall.

Compressors

Compressor motors must be cooled during their operation; this is accomplished by the use of either an oil- or an air-cooled system (Figs. 3.4–3.6).[1,3,4] If the compressor has an oil-cooled motor then the oil will need to be maintained at a certain level and periodically changed to maximize the life of the motor.[1,3,4] Air-cooled motors, on the other hand, do not require oil maintenance and therefore have the advantage that oil from the motor cannot get into the handpieces and air-lines.[3,4] Oil residue in the handpieces can shorten the life of the handpiece as well as interfering with bonding and curing of some restorative compounds.[3,4]

The compressor will generate some level of noise output depending on the size and capabilities of the compressor.[1,3,4] Compressors that are larger and capable of running more than one dental delivery unit may be housed in an area away from the dental operatory to prevent excessive noise levels.[1,3,4]

Compressors also require the air storage tank to be drained of any condensation daily.[1,3,4] The air tank will fill up with water over time, reducing the availability of space to compress air, thus causing the motor to turn on frequently.[1,3,4] Overworking the motor could eventually cause its failure due to overheating.[1,3,4]

Motor-Driven Units

Electric motor-driven units are also available for use as a high- or low-speed alternative for handpieces.[1,4] In general, the capabilities of these are limited to a speed range

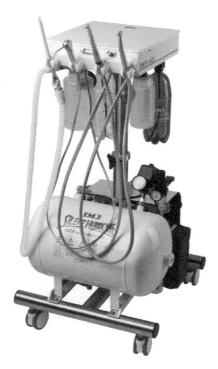

Figure 3.4   iM3® Elite with silent hurricane compressor (Courtesy of iM3 Inc. "The Veterinary Dental Company").

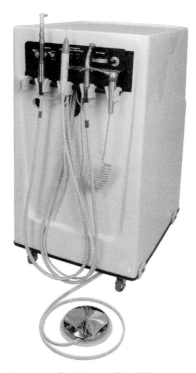

Figure 3.5   Ultima dental unit (Courtesy of MAI Animal Health).

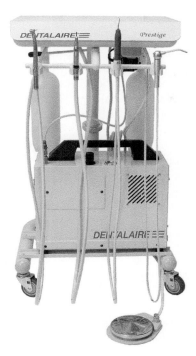

Figure 3.6   Dentalaire Prestige dental delivery unit (Courtesy of Dentalaire).

of 3000–30,000 rpm, which is much slower than the air-driven units.[4] The advantage of these units is that they are small, very portable, and less expensive and offer more torque than the air-driven units.[4]

Some disadvantages are as follows:

- The inability to run water through the handpieces to cool the dental tissues and prevent hyperthermic damage. Water must be dripped by someone from a syringe continuously while teeth are being sectioned.[1,4]
- The motor and handpieces may not be capable of a demanding, constant workload without breaking down.[4]
- The slower rotational speeds make sectioning of larger teeth and other procedures more difficult to accomplish due to the high torque causing excessive movement of the tip, leading to instability during use.[4]

Summary of Dental Delivery Units

Most dental delivery units operate with a rheostat or foot pedal to engage or control each handpiece when the handpiece is removed from its specific cradle on the unit.

Dental delivery units must fit in the dental operatory along with other equipment, offer all of the features and benefits that are needed, have minimal maintenance and repair needs, offer minimum noise levels and be adaptable in position to accommodate both right- and left-handed operators.

Dental Handpieces

Handpieces are the operational part of the dental unit that rests in the operator's hand. Each handpiece facilitates the use of either rotational or ultrasonic forces driven by compressed air, gases, or electricity to maximize the effectiveness of certain dental burs, disks, polishing angles, scaler tips, and other instruments, to section, change the shape or contour of tooth or bone, and to clean, polish, or finish the final tooth structure during a procedure.[1-4]

Each handpiece connects to individual air and water-lines that run from the central dental unit to the handpiece.

The four most commonly used handpieces are:

- High-speed handpiece
- Low-speed handpiece
- Three-way air–water syringe
- Ultrasonic scaler

High-Speed Handpiece

High-speed handpieces rotate at up to 400,000 rpm with low torque (Fig. 3.7).[1-4] A turbine contained in the working end of the handpiece uses friction grip (FG) burs.[1-4]

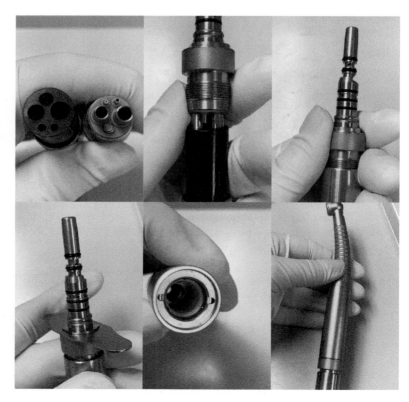

Figure 3.7   Assembly of high-speed dental handpiece. (Courtesy of Pawsitive Dental Education LLC).

These burs are used when sectioning teeth, removing alveolar bone, alveoloplasty, endodontic access, cavity preparation, and other procedures.[1-4] High-speed handpieces use low torque and therefore may stall out if excessive pressure is applied to the tooth or bone with the rotating bur by the operator's hand.[2]

Care of the high-speed handpiece

Remember to never run a high-speed handpiece without a bur or "blank" inserted in the chuck; this may cause the chuck to be damaged.[1,3,4]

High-speed burs do occasionally "stall" due to their lower torque forces; this prevents the possibility of shattering the tooth or other bone being cut or altered.[2,3]

The speed at which the high-speed handpiece's bur rotates is controlled by the dental unit's rheostat or foot pedal. It is essential that the handpiece is running at maximum speed when the bur touches the surface of the tooth or bone.

Water supplied to the cutting end of the bur provides cooling at these higher speeds, preventing thermal damage to the tooth and bone.[1-4]

High-speed handpieces require daily maintenance to ensure their longevity and optimum usefulness (Fig. 3.8).[1-4] Cleaning and conditioning spray specially formulated for the handpiece should be placed in the smaller of the two holes on the bottom of the handpiece daily after use, and then the handpiece run with a "blank" or bur for several seconds to disperse the lubricant through the handpiece.[1,3-5]

To prevent the spread of disease, these handpieces should be cleaned, lubricated, and autoclaved in between patients.[1,2,5] Consult the manufacturer's directions for specific maintenance on the handpiece that you need to maintain. Bleaching solution must never be run through a high-speed handpiece, only through the water-lines of the unit if directed by the manufacturer.

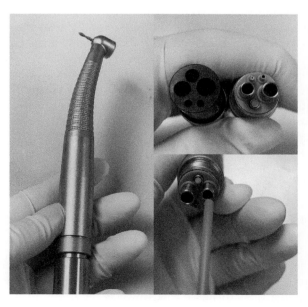

Figure 3.8 High-speed handpiece maintenance (Courtesy of Pawsitive Dental Education LLC).

Fiber optics

Some high-speed handpieces, as well as ultrasonic scalers, are equipped with fiber optic light sources that are very useful in visualization of the working area while the handpiece is in use (see web content: Fig. 3.9W). Extra light bulbs should be on hand for replacement as needed.

High-speed dental burs

Dental burs come in different lengths, from standard lengths (S) to surgical length (SL) shanks, with various diameters and lengths to the cutting end.[1-4] High-speed burs are changed using a push-button or key system to release or engage the chuck's hold on the bur. The dental bur must be fully inserted and locked in place when used (see web content: Fig. 3.10W).

These burs are typically made of carbide steel and are for use on one patient only because the bur becomes dull fairly quickly. If they are reused, the turbine, which is housed in the head of the high-speed handpiece, becomes stressed due to the operator placing more pressure on the bur's shank while attempting to section tooth or remove bone; this force will reduce the life span of the turbine.

Low-Speed Handpiece

Primarily used for polishing the tooth's surface after ultrasonic and hand scaling procedures, these handpieces come in different styles, such as traditional, operative, restorative, and hygiene (see web content: Figs. 3.11W and 3.12W). Attachments fit with either an E-type, which is a quick release, pull-off or push-on type of attachment, or the Doriot-type which has a twist locking mechanism.[3] Low-speed handpieces often have a control to adjust the rotation of the attachment from forward to neutral to reverse, located near the connection with the air-drive line> The speed on the dental delivery unit is adjusted by a foot pedal. Operational speed for polishing should be adjusted to between 2000 and 4000 rpm. Use of the appropriate rotational speed for polishing prevents splatter of the prophy paste and increases handpiece control.

Low-speed handpieces should not be used for cutting bone. Although their higher torque makes it less likely that the bur will stop rotating during the procedure, they will take more time to do the job, thus creating more heat due to friction.[1-3] Increased friction can cause tooth, tissue, or bone to heat up, due to the lack of water to rinse and cool the area.[1-4]

Low-speed attachments

Prophy angles
Before using the low-speed handpiece to "polish" teeth at the end of a dental cleaning procedure, you will need to attach a disposable oscillating or rotating prophy angle to the Doriot-type handpiece. Attaching the prophy angle is done by turning the ring near the open end of the handpiece which allows placement of the prophy angle's post into the handpiece. Once fully inserted, the post of the prophy angle is locked in by turning the adjustable ring towards the newly installed plastic angle. Metal reusable prophy angles are also available but do require maintenance and,

in general, do not oscillate.[1,2] Angles that have a circular rotation can also grab long hairs and wrap them around the prophy angle, causing trauma to the patient as well as causing the operator to have to stop and unwrap the hair.[1-4] Plastic debris from the post of the disposable prophy angle can accumulate in the handpiece's opening. This debris can be easily cleaned out using a hypodermic needle inserted into the central hole where the plastic drive post would be inserted, reaming out the accumulation, and then shaking it out of the handpiece's opening by inverting the handpiece. Do this weekly to prevent blockage (see web content: Fig. 3.13W).

Contra-angles

With low-speed handpieces a contra-angle attachment can be used to reduce or increase the speed at which the tip rotates and to give a greater than 90-degree angle of access during restorations of posterior teeth.[2-4] This is useful when procedures such as endodontic preparations are to be performed or when the angulations need to be changed to give greater access.[3,4] A reversed direction of rotation can also be used in certain procedures to "back-out" of endodontic access sites.[3,4]

The most common "step-up" contra-angle is the 4:1, which would increase the speed from 20,000 to 80,000 rpm, and a "step-down" angle would be the 10:1 reduction gear.[3,4] Right-angle (RA) burs, which are larger than the high-speed handpiece burs and have a "latch-type" attachment, are required to use these contra-angle attachments.[3] Another type of contra-angle is the Doriot-type, which takes a type of bur labeled as HP. These are even longer and bigger in diameter than the right-angle burs.[3]

Three-Way Air–Water Syringe

The three-way air and water syringe operates by using pressurized air in the compressor's tank. One button produces a stream of water, one produces pressurized air, and both used together supplies a mixture of distilled water and air to the dentition. A mixture of pressurized air and water can be helpful to rinse away debris and polishing paste. Gently drying dental surfaces during the procedure can help to disclose residual tartar on the enamel as well.

Ultrasonic Scalers

Powered ultrasonic scaling units are designed to help the practitioner perform a professional dental cleaning by using ultrasonic forces to aid in the removal of plaque and calculus from the dental surfaces both supra- and subgingivally.[1-4] Ultrasonic scaling can shorten the cleaning time dramatically, thus decreasing patient anesthetic times.[1-4] A pressurized water source is necessary to irrigate and cool the working tip of the instrument.[1-4] Ultrasonic scalers can be integrated into the dental unit itself or can be independent. Independently operating units require a pressurized water supply from a small water tank that must be pumped by hand before use.

Ultrasonic scalers come in two different configurations: magnetostrictive, which utilizes a ferrite rod or ferromagnetic stack, or piezoelectric.[1-4] When alternating current (AC) is applied, a magnetic field is created around either the ferromagnetic insert or ferrite rod in the magnetostrictive handpiece or quartz crystal disks in the piezoelectric handpiece. Specific inserts or tips then vibrate in a certain predictable pattern.[1-4]

Water flow adjustments

Water flowing through the handpiece creates tiny vacuum bubbles (cavitation) as it flows along the tip of the handpiece. The micro-movement of the tip to the tooth's surface facilitates the removal of plaque and calculus.[1-4] It is imperative that the water supply is adjusted correctly to create a misty spray that projects off the last 3 mm of the tip outward.[1-4]

Unit frequency

Frequency is a term used to indicate the number of times the tip of the scaler completes a single pattern per second (cycles per second or hertz [Hz]).[1-3] The frequencies of different ultrasonic scalers can range from 18,000 to 45,000 Hz.[1-3]

Power settings

It is important to note that the power control on the scaler is used to adjust the distance that the tip travels (amplitude) in its specific pattern: linear (piezoelectric), elliptical or figure-of-eight (magnetostrictive metal strips), elliptical (ferrite rod), and that certain types of tips are more or less active on specific sides.[2,3]

Ultrasonic scaler tips and inserts

Magnetostrictive inserts and tips

The ferromagnetic stack comprises a working end attached to a base of strips of laminated nickel which are attached at the bottom with solder (see web content: Fig. 3.14W).[1-4] These inserts need to be monitored very closely for any sign of separation or fracture of the strips of nickel. If the attachment of the welding has broken down at the end, the strips become ineffective.[1-4] The insert should be placed in the handpiece after the handpiece has been filled with water from the dental unit.[1] Insert by gently pushing the appropriate insert into the handle. To remove after use, twist slightly and pull.[1]

One disadvantage of having scalers that require only special inserts of a specific frequency is that they are not necessarily interchangeable with all types of magnetostrictive scaler models.[1,4] You must purchase the frequency of ultrasonic scaler insert that is compatible with the scaler that you are using. A 25 kHz scaler insert and a 30 kHz insert differ in the length of stack and the number of vibrations per second that they are capable of producing.[1,3,4]

Ferrite rod inserts are inserted with the handpiece drained of water. Failure to empty the handpiece before insertion of the ferrite rod can result in the fracture of the tip.[1,4] Care should be taken to ensure that the rod insert is not dropped because they are very fragile.[4]

Piezoelectric tips

Piezoelectric units offer small metal tip options that are attached and removed by using a small wrench specific to the unit's design (see web content: Fig. 3.15W). Be very careful not to over-tighten the tip; this can strip out the threads.[1-4] Working at a frequency of 25,000–45,000 Hz in a linear pattern, the tip moves in a wide amplitude of up to 0.2 mm. Piezoelectric tips are also cooled by the continuous water flowing along the tip.[1-4]

General ultrasonic tip function

Supra- and subgingival scaler tips are not the same; supragingival tips can only be used on the crown's surface, not below the gingival margin.[1-4] Subgingival tips are longer and thinner, allowing the water to flow to the end of the tip to facilitate proper cooling and lavage on the root's surface.[2]

Magnetostrictive stack tips are active on all sides and along the last 5–7 mm of the tip, whereas the ferrite rod tips are active along and around the whole 12 mm of the tip; piezoelectric tips are active on the terminal 3 mm only.[2] Piezoelectric tips potentially could be less damaging to the tooth when appropriately used, due to reduced thermal production (see web content: Fig. 3.16W).[1]

Tip care and maintenance

When using any ultrasonic scaler, attention must be paid to the length of the working end.[1-4] Before use, always measure the tip's length on the manufacturer's tip card. Even a 1 mm loss of length will dramatically (by 25%) reduce the effectiveness of the tip.[1-4] When tips have lost 2 mm of their length they should be replaced due to loss of 50% of their efficacy.[1-4]

All ultrasonic tips should be cleaned and autoclaved between uses and kept sterile until ready to use in order to prevent patient cross-contamination.[4,5]

Summary of Power Equipment

All members of the veterinary dental team should take time to become educated and clear about the use and maintenance of all power equipment used in the dental operatory.[5] Safe use of the equipment on patients depends on careful cleaning, sterilization, maintenance, repair, and correct application procedures and techniques. Members of the team should read the manufacturer's directions and recommendations and follow these explicitly for best results.

Dental Tables and Chairs

A table for the patient undergoing dental care is a required item in veterinary dentistry. Without this surface, we would not be able to perform the procedures correctly. Unfortunately, we cannot have our animal patients in a comfortable chair that reclines as in the human dental operatory, so veterinarians have used many different types of surfaces over the years to accommodate our patients. We will discuss how the dental table has evolved over the years, how ergonomics for the dental operator has taken the forefront in achieving a more comfortable posture for the dental team, and the differences between using a "wet" table and a "dry" table.

Tables available are either permanently fixed or mobile, with various features:

- Dry table with a flat countertop surface, with or without a basin at the working end
- Wet, tub-like table with a flat stationary surface
- Dry table with adjustable slope and height, with or without a basin system at the working end to catch water and fluids. Some have a surface that is adjustable,

with sides that can be raised independently to provide lateral support for a patient in dorsal recumbency. This type resembles a standard surgical table
■ Wet free-standing table with hydraulic lift to raise the patient from near floor level to comfortable working level for the operator
■ Wet or dry free-standing lift table with integrated dental unit and compressor with the capacity to add accessories

Dry Tables

 Dry tables can either be fixed or mobile (see web content: Figs. 3.17W and 3.18W).

Fixed tables

A fixed dry table may be a treatment table that is utilized for dentistry. It is usually attached to a wall, countertop, or cabinet. It may have an area at the working end where the operator can place their legs under the edge of the table while working in a sitting position.[2,3] Some fixed tables do not allow space for a person to sit comfortably at the working end due to the lack of leg room under the table, so the operator may have to work in a standing position.

Mobile or non-fixed table

A non-fixed table may be a metal (stainless steel) surgical type table on wheels or a "lift" table with the ability for height adjustment so that the veterinary professional can sit comfortably. Lift tables usually have a foot pedal or other switch to raise or lower the table as necessary, thus not requiring the dental operator to lift heavy patients to tabletop height.

Wet Tables

Wet dental tables have a water supply plumbed in and a tub or basin area to collect the excess water and debris that accumulate when dental procedures are being performed (see web content: Fig. 3.19W). Excess water and debris can fall into the tub or basin below the patient's head or body and then be cleaned away quickly after the procedure with the water supply hose and a spray nozzle that is integrated into the plumbing of the table. Keeping the patient clean, free of debris, and dry is vital to help prevent hypothermia due to the cooling effects of water from the spray of the ultrasonic scaler, high-speed handpiece, or air–water syringe on the dental delivery unit.[6,7] Having the tub or basin under the patient allows the operator to rinse away debris, polish paste, and blood from the patient's mouth without soaking the head and coat with water. The downside to a wet-tub table is the potential for loss of the patient's body heat due to the open area under the patient's body if it is not well insulated by active warming devices and towels or blankets.

If the table has a slope toward the working end where the patient's head is positioned it will help to drain any water and debris from the patient's oral cavity into the basin or tub.

Contemporary dental tables that have a basin or tub and water availability often also have the ability to lift the patient and adjust the working height to suit the operator's needs. Height adjustment helps to ensure that the operator is sitting comfortably and using a more ergonomic posture to help prevent work-related injuries to back, neck, and arms.

Table Recommendations

Dental patient tables should be between 60 and 84 inches (1.5–2 m) in length and around 24–30 inches (60–76 cm) in width. If the table is stationary, a good working height is 36 inches (91 cm) to allow the operator to sit comfortably. If the height is adjustable, the operator can adjust this as necessary. Adjustable-height tables are always preferred to allow for ease of use for any operator and any sized companion animal. Other things to consider are: Does the table provide patient warming? Is the table going to wick heat away from the patient? Does the table have surfaces that are easily cleaned and disinfected? The cost of the table? How versatile is this table with different sized patients? Can you attach anesthesia equipment, monitoring equipment, procedure trays, and other needed items to the table to keep clutter off the floor space? How easy is it to move the table to adjust the height or position as needed?

The area where dental procedures are performed is often part of a busy treatment room area. However, dental departments of the future should be dedicated spaces designed with room to work comfortably and safely. Features such as waste anesthetic gas removal, room air circulation, temperature controls, lighting, floor surfaces, cabinetry, and storage all make a difference in how well the dental operatory functions. Considerations such as ensuring dental radiographs can be obtained without exposing those around the area to radiation should be a part of the dental operatory planning procedures.

Care and Use

Working tables should be maintained in a clean and disinfected state. Organic debris should be thoroughly removed and the top surface disinfected. The contact time of any disinfectant is critical to ensure that microorganisms are killed. Working parts, such as those in mobile, lift, or wet tables, should be maintained according to the manufacturer's instructions to provide a functioning table for as long as possible.

Dental Chairs

Several factors should be considered when deciding which dental chair is best for you (see web content: Fig. 3.20W). Everything from the height adjustment, to what kind of lumbar support it may have, to the tilt and adjustability of the seat itself are important. Chairs designed primarily for use in the dental operatory are usually best as they are made for prolonged use by the operator performing dentistry. There is a need for significant adjustability due to differences in the size of personnel and different species of veterinary patients, often with extreme variations in patient size. Ideally, the chair should feel comfortable to you, allow you to maintain a firm placement of your feet, either on a ring around the base or on the floor itself. You should be sitting high enough that your forearms are parallel to the floor when at table height, with your upper arms in alignment with your torso. The table should adjust to your comfortable seated height. If all of these circumstances do not coordinate well, the operator usually has to accommodate the mismatch by adjusting their body, and this can lead to strains and pains that could develop into permanent disabilities over time.

Organizing the Dental Operatory

Some primary considerations need to be met to have a dental operatory that is functional, organized, and efficient. Looking at the size of your space, you want to ensure that you can comfortably work with the patient on the table, allowing room for all of the equipment and instruments during a procedure, and space to freely move in and out of the 6 foot (2 m) zone around the patient's head while dental radiographs are obtained.

All of the instrumentation used during the procedure, including the dental delivery unit, should be located on the dominant side of the operator.

The dental team member who is providing dedicated patient monitoring should have easy access to the patient, anesthetic machine, monitors, warming devices, and miscellaneous supplies needed for patient care.

Floor space should be kept free of tripping hazards, and extra equipment should not be stored or left in the operatory.

Regular assessments of the equipment, instruments, tables, and all items in the dental operatory should be performed to ensure that the working area is in good order and functioning well.

Personal Protection

Types of Hazards

In the veterinary profession, there are three types of hazards that one must be aware of during employment: physical hazards, chemical hazards, and biologic hazards.

Physical hazards

These include injuries resulting from patient handling, such as bites and scratches or lifting injuries, radiation exposure, excessive noise levels, slip or trip and fall types of accidents, repetitive motion injuries, and cumulative trauma disorders, poor ergonomic practices, injury due to handling of sharp dental instruments, needles or other equipment.[2-4]

Chemical hazards

These include exposure to harmful chemicals through skin or mucous membrane contact, inhalation, or other exposures either chronic or acute.[2-4] Some commonly found chemical hazards in the dental operatory include the following:

- Anesthetic gases
- Chemicals to develop and fix dental X-ray film

- Free mercury found in dental amalgams
- Concentrated chemical disinfectants
- Acids, resins, and catalysts from dental restoratives
- Sodium hypochlorite

Biologic hazards

These come from the patient's mouth and body as well as potentially from humans working in the operatory. Potentially infectious or harmful bacteria, viruses, fungi, spores, or toxins can be inhaled, ingested, or absorbed through mucous membranes, such as those of the eyes or mouth, or cuts or scratches in the skin barrier from contaminated equipment and instruments. Aerosolization of harmful bacteria occurs when performing dental procedures, and bacteria-laden debris can be propelled into the operator's eyes and potentially cause severe consequences to the vision and eye health. Any contact with the patient's biological matter, such as blood or saliva, or with another operator's bodily fluids in the case of injury could transmit disease and infections.

The Occupational Safety and Health Administration (OSHA), along with the National Institute for Occupational Safety and Health (NIOSH) and the Centers for Disease Control (CDC), provide employers and employees with guidelines to regulate safety in the workplace through enforcement of the Hazard Communication Standard.

Employer Responsibilities

Employer responsibilities include provision of the following:

- Access to a comprehensive Material Safety Data Sheet (MSDS) file so that all employees can educate themselves on what chemical hazards are possible and how to respond if there is a chemical accident
- Initial and ongoing training on safety in the workplace
- Personal protective equipment (PPE) so that employees can wear these items to protect themselves from potential acute or cumulative injury
- A safe and maintained work area for the employee free of known physical hazards
- Training, equipment manuals, and a maintenance protocol for each piece of equipment that the employee will be required to use

Employee Responsibilities

Employees are responsible for:

- Reading and understanding MSDS files that are made available in the hospital
- Wearing the required PPE during procedures
- Knowing how to use the eyewash station
- Becoming familiar with any equipment that will be used and knowing safety procedures with that equipment
- Attending all regular safety meetings and training sessions

CHAPTER 3

The above items are just some of the responsibilities that employers and employees both must assume to work toward safety in the veterinary hospital collectively.

Personal Protective Equipment (PPE)

Gloves

Gloves must be worn at all times to protect the operator from skin exposure to biological and chemical contamination through open wounds, micro-abrasions, or chemical contact injury.[2] Gloves offer protection from repeated exposure to common chemicals and solutions used when practicing dentistry. Some of these solutions could potentially harm the liver or kidneys with repeated exposure and could be potential carcinogens.[2]

Gloves should always be worn over freshly washed hands.[2] Proper handwashing techniques prevent bacteria residing on our skin from causing infection in the case of a puncture or abrasion on the skin.

Gloves play a dual role in that they also help prevent cross-contamination from one patient to another with biological or chemical exposures to the glove's surface.[2]

Gloves should be right and left specific to avoid incorrect fit, which could cause fatigue and injury to the small joints in the hands over time.[2] They should neither be too tight fitting nor too loose.[2] Surgical gloves that are sized by number may be a good choice if right- and left-handed exam gloves are unavailable (see web content: Fig. 3.21W). Avoid latex gloves and powdered gloves if you have allergies to these materials.[2]

Eye protection

Everyone in the dental operatory area must wear safety glasses. When using instruments or an ultrasonic scaler, particles such as tartar or tooth pieces or broken metal burs when using a high-speed handpiece do become airborne and can cause eye injury or infection.[1-4] Sprays of chemicals and acid-etching materials can also inflict serious harm to eyes.[2]

Possible options include typical safety glasses, plastic shields that cover the eyes extending upward from face masks, ocular protection provided by eye loupes that magnify the operatory field, or special prescription safety glasses made for specific users.[2-5]

During light-curing of composites or resins, specially made glasses that have a filter should be worn. Do not look directly at the light emitted by the curing device because these lights can cause permanent retinal damage.[2]

Face masks

A mask covering the nose and mouth should be worn during all dental procedures by all personnel working within a 3–4 foot (1–1.2 m) radius of the patient. Respiratory protection prevents inhalation of bacteria and other biological contaminants.[2] The mask should fit well and not be too loose; an ill-fitting mask can allow contaminants in and will also cause fogging of safety eyewear. Surgical masks are often used, but masks that are made specifically for respiratory protection are more effective at blocking potentially hazardous material.[2,3]

Protective clothing and caps

Wearing a dental operatory gown or jacket and a surgical hat will protect the user from bacterial contamination of work clothing and hair that could be carried out of the dental area and contaminate other hospital areas or patients (see web content: Fig. 3.22W).

Hearing protection

The use of high-speed handpieces, ultrasonic scalers, low-speed handpieces, model trimmers, vibrators, and suction units can result in levels of noise that are high enough, over time, to cause hearing loss.[3] Operators of such equipment or those in the dental operatory should wear hearing protection during the procedures to minimize this risk.[4] Common earplugs should help prevent damage due to these high-decibel noises.[3]

Dosimetry badges and radiation safety

A dosimetry badge provides ongoing monitoring of employee exposure to radiation. The dental operator should always wear their dosimetry badge when obtaining dental radiographs. Never stand within 6 feet (2 m) of the X-ray tube head if unprotected by a lead apron. Never hold the sensor or phosphor plate in the mouth of a patient with or without lead gloves. A lead plate placed under the patient's head during X-rays can help prevent excess scatter radiation.

Ergonomics

The word ergonomics originates from the Greek words *ergon*, meaning work, and *nomos*, meaning natural laws. The Polish researcher Professor Wojciech Jastrzebowski first used the word to describe his theories in 1857.[6] Since then, many organizations have been set up throughout the world to study and focus on the development of ergonomic equipment, methods, and systems. The goal is to achieve optimal performance of work through awareness of human anatomy, physiology, and psychology and to allow safe, effective, comfortable, and productive work to take place.[8–10]

Ergonomics as it pertains to veterinary dentistry is in the early stages of development and has not become a consistent practice.[1,8,10] Because of this, the dental team should be acutely aware of ergonomic principles and practices and consider them when choosing equipment for the dental operatory.

Work-Related Musculoskeletal Disorders

Workplace injuries, both acute and chronic, result in loss of working time and have a substantial impact on a veterinary hospital's financial health.

Cumulative Trauma or Repetitive Strain Disorders

Repetitive motions, such as those required by veterinary dentistry, utilize the small muscles and joints in your hands and wrists along with the larger muscles and joints of the upper body, including shoulders, neck or back. Over time this motion can lead to strains due to tasks being repeated to the point of fatigue and then to muscular exhaustion.[3] Such cumulative trauma can eventually result in a chronic disorder, which, if not allowed to heal, can lead to permanent changes in those joints, nerves, vasculature, and muscles.[6] Many disorders are caused by repetitive movements, such as carpal tunnel syndrome (affects the median nerve in the wrist and hand), Guyon's canal syndrome (ulnar nerve entrapment at the wrist), cubital tunnel syndrome (ulnar nerve compression at the elbow), and thoracic outlet syndrome (neurovascular compression affecting the shoulder, arm, and hand). These and many other chronic stress disorders are mostly preventable using ergonomic principles.[3–5]

Symptoms of such repetitive motion injuries will often be similar in nature and a physician should always be consulted if an injury is suspected.[4] Prevention of injury is of utmost importance due to the nature of dentistry.

Participatory Ergonomics – Finding Solutions

All team members should be involved in recognizing ergonomic hazards in the workplace and should be encouraged to collectively come up with strategies and solutions. Time management also plays a role with regard to repetitive motion injuries.

Ergonomics should be considered when purchasing hand instrumentation as well as power equipment. Larger, lighter handled instruments should be used whenever possible to prevent tight gripping of small items and team members should be trained in use of a correct neutral arm, wrist, and sitting posture.[2,4] Changing motions or actions frequently to prevent continued stress to certain muscle groups can also help to prevent repetitive strain injury.[4]

Careful attention to the use of the correct instrument for the task, making sure the instrument is sharp, not damaged, and held with a neutral wrist posture will reduce the risk of a disorder.[4]

Utilizing power instrumentation whenever possible will decrease the strain of excessive use of hand instruments alone.[2,4]

Convenient placement of equipment and items most often used in the dental operatory will reduce the need for twisting and reaching movements, further reducing strain on the body during procedures.

The use of "line of sight" lighting, where the light line is parallel to the direction of your sight, such as a fiber optic or direct halogen light mounted on a headband or magnification loupes/glasses will decrease the tilting of the head forward. Ensuring that the entire working area can be visualized easily will significantly reduce injuries sustained due to improper posture, leaning over the patient and table, and raising the elbows above the working area to accomplish tasks (see web content: Figs. 3.23W, 3.24W, and 3.25W).[6,8,11]

Using adjustable tables and ergonomic seating can significantly increase operator comfort during procedural work.

References

1. Holmstrom, SE. 2019. Dental instruments and equipment. In *Veterinary Dentistry: A Team Approach*, 3rd edn (ed. SE Holmstrom). St. Louis, MO:

Elsevier, pp. 73–110; Holmstrom, SE, Holmstrom LA. 2019. Personal safety and ergonomics. In *Veterinary Dentistry: a Team Approach*, 3rd edn (ed. SE Holmstrom). St. Louis, MO: Elsevier, pp. 111–124.

2. Niemiec, BA. 2013. *Veterinary Periodontology*. Ames, IA: Wiley Blackwell.

3. Holmstrom, SE, Fitch, PF, Eisner, ER. 2004. *Dental equipment and care. In Veterinary Dental Techniques for the Small Animal Practitioner*, 3rd edn. Philadelphia, PA: Elsevier, chapter 2.

4. Bellows, J. *Small Animal Dental Equipment, Materials and Techniques: A Primer*, 2nd edn. Ames, IA: Wiley Blackwell, 2019.

5. Bellows, J, Berg, ML, Dennis S et al. 2019. *AAHA Dental Care Guidelines for Dogs and Cats*. https://www.aaha.org/globalassets/02-guidelines/dental/aaha_dental_guidelines.pdf (accessed March 2020).

6. Stepaniuk, K, Brock, N. 2008. Hypothermia and thermoregulation during anesthesia for the dental and oral surgery patient. *Journal of Veterinary Dentistry* 25:279–283.

7. Pollack-Simon, R. 2002. *All the Right Moves*. Tulsa, OK: Penn Well.

8. Aller, MS. 2005. Personal safety and ergonomics in the dental operatory. *Journal of Veterinary Dentistry* 22:124–130.

9. Murphy, DC. 1998. *Ergonomics and the Dental Care Worker*. Washington, DC: American Public Health Association.

10. DeForge, DH. 2002. Physical ergonomics in veterinary dentistry. *Journal of Veterinary Dentistry* 19:196–200.

11. Chang, BJ. 2002. *Guidelines for Selecting Ergonomically Correct Surgical Telescope Systems*. Chesterland, OH: Academy of Dental Therapeutics and Stomatology.

Anesthesia and the Dental Patient

Annie Mills, LVT, VTS (Dentistry)

Learning Objectives

- Facilitate a successful anesthetic event from induction to recovery
- Understand pain and its effects on the dental patient, and to implement an effective pain management protocol
- Choose a safe and effective anesthetic protocol
- Facilitate a successful anesthetic event for the dental patient from induction to recovery
- Understand pain and its effects on the dental patient
- Formulate and implement an effective pain management protocol

Small Animal Dental Procedures for Veterinary Technicians and Nurses, Second Edition.
Edited by Jeanne R. Perrone.
© 2021 John Wiley & Sons, Inc. Published 2021 by John Wiley & Sons, Inc.

Introduction

The following will be an in-depth discussion of anesthetic equipment, monitoring devices, and pain management techniques. The reader should become familiar with this information to implement the techniques in everyday practice.

Numerous marketing surveys have shown that the number one reason pet owners decline professional dental care is not a financial one, but because of their fear of anesthesia.[1] Many patients may suffer needlessly with periodontal disease because of this fear and the reluctance of the owner to consent to a professional dental cleaning procedure. It is essential that pet owners are educated by the veterinary team and explain that the benefits of professional dental care and treatment far outweigh the risks of anesthesia. It is also the role of the veterinary team to alleviate the pet owners' fears by minimizing anesthetic risks and becoming proficient in providing effective and safe anesthesia for the dental patient. This is accomplished by becoming well versed in anesthetic protocols and techniques and through comprehensive monitoring techniques. The pain management protocol is also an essential component in the anesthetic plan to aid in the overall success of the dental patient's treatment and recovery. By encompassing all pain pathways, using preemptive pain management, and addressing postoperative pain, the veterinary team can "cover all the bases" of the dental patient's pain relief.

Anesthesia for the Dental Patient

The keys to the success of any anesthetic event lie in the knowledge and preparedness of the veterinary team, the reliability of the anesthetic equipment, and diligent monitoring throughout the entire event. The following sections will discuss anesthetic protocols available to veterinary professionals, and the anesthetic equipment required to maintain and monitor a safe and effective anesthetic plane.

Presurgical Assessment

Before beginning any anesthetic procedure, the veterinary team must evaluate and anticipate the needs of the patient based on a variety of criteria that include, but are not limited to, age, breed, weight, the procedure being performed, and any physiological conditions associated with the patient. A physical exam, a thorough history, and a comprehensive preanesthetic diagnostic workup should be performed before any anesthetic procedure. The most common tests in a preanesthetic workup include a complete blood count to rule out any anemias and bacterial or viral infections, a full chemistry panel, electrolyte panel, and urinalysis. These tests can indicate the normal or abnormal function of the major organs. An electrocardiogram (ECG) before anesthesia is important to rule out any abnormal arrhythmias. Chest radiographs may be recommended as an additional preanesthetic screening test for older patients and those with oral masses suspect of neoplasia. For any patient where there is a suspicion of cardiac disease (coughing, prolonged capillary refill time, murmur, pulse deficits), a cardiac workup is indicated before initiating dental procedures.

Some anesthetic protocols can be detrimental to a patient with early kidney or liver disease or a patient with cardiac abnormalities. The anesthetic protocol should be tailored to the patient based on the previous criteria and all preanesthetic diag-nostic data. A thorough preanesthetic evaluation is a vital first step in reducing the risk of anesthesia for the dental patient. In this regard, fractious pets who present to veterinary hospitals require special consideration.

Premedicants

Premedication is important to the anesthetic regimen for several reasons. The major-ity of veterinary patients are in a heightened state of fear after being admitted into the hospital for a dental procedure. A sedative, because of its calming effect, reduces their stress level and facilitates the preoperative preparation of the patient. During the procedure, an opioid premedication allows the anesthetist to use a lower rate of inhalant anesthesia due to its analgesic properties. This will be discussed more thor-oughly later in this chapter. There are many premedication drug combinations avail-able to the veterinary anesthetist. The key is deciding which regimen to choose for a particular patient. As previously stated, protocols should be chosen based on the patient's information (age, breed, etc.), the data gathered during the preoperative workup, the physical exam, and the temperament of the patient. Any preexisting conditions should also be considered when choosing the drug protocol. It is impor-tant to note that anesthesia in the dental patient, in many instances, will involve anesthesia for the geriatric patient as well, since these two groups often overlap. Although advanced age is not a disease in itself, it can bring about physiological changes in the patient that must be considered before the anesthetic procedure (Table 4.1).

Induction Agents and Inhalants

As with premedications, there are also numerous choices in induction agents and these should be chosen carefully based on the patient's needs. The goal here is to induce the patient to the point of sedation so that an endotracheal tube may be placed. This will then facilitate the use of an inhalant anesthetic to continue and maintain a safe anesthetic plane. A ketamine and diazepam combination is a reliable and fairly safe protocol; however, propofol is becoming more widely used because it is poorly absorbed by the major organs and has a short recovery time. These induc-tion agents should be administered carefully and only "to effect" in order to insert an endotracheal tube. Modern inhalants (including isoflurane and sevoflurane) are preferred because of their low solubility. They permit a rapid induction and recovery, as well as allowing the anesthetic plane to be adjusted as needed. They do not depend on metabolism to any significant degree for removal from the body.

Anesthetic Equipment

Modern anesthetic machines and breathing systems control the delivery of inhalant anesthetics and oxygen and eliminate waste gases from the environment of the oper-ating room.[2] The anesthetic machine is equipped with a vaporizer to deliver a mix-ture of inhalant anesthetic and oxygen to the patient at a controlled rate (Fig. 4.1).

CHAPTER 4

Table 4.1   Table of premedication protocols

Drug	Class of drug	Dose if used in combination	Advantages	Disadvantages
Acepromazine	Phenothiazine	Dog: 0.005– 0.060 mg/kg Cat: 0.04– 0.10 mg/kg	Excellent sedation when used in combination with an opioid	No analgesic effects
Butorphanol	Opioid	Dog: 0.1–0.4 mg/kg Cat: 0.1–0.4 mg/kg	Analgesic properties	Very short duration of analgesic effects
Morphine	Reversible opioid	Dog: 0.5–1 mg/kg Cat: 0.5–1 mg/kg	Potent analgesic properties	Hypersensitivity in cats; can cause bradycardia and respiratory depression
Hydromophone	Reversible opioid	Dog: 0.10–0.20 mg/kg Cat: 0.10–0.20 mg/kg	Potent analgesic properties	Can cause bradycardia and respiratory depression
Oxymorphone	Reversible opioid	Dog: 0.05–0.10 mg/kg Cat: 0.05–0.10 mg/kg	Potent analgesic properties	Can cause bradycardia and respiratory depression, noise sensitivity
Fentanyl	Reversible opioid	Dog: 0.005–0.010 mg/kg Cat: 0.005–0.10 mg/kg	Potent analgesic properties	Can cause bradycardia and respiratory depression
Medetomidine	Alpha-2 agonist	Dog: 0.002–0.40 mg/kg Cat: 0.002–0.40 mg/kg	Potent analgesic properties, reversible	Can cause bradycardia
Buprenorphine	Synthetic opiate	Dog: 0.10–0.40 mg/kg Cat: 0.10–0.40 mg/kg	Undesirable effects are rare	Limited reversibility

The anesthetic machine should be assessed at the beginning of the day before any anesthetic procedures. All parts of the machine should be closely examined for any defects; the oxygen and anesthetic inhalant levels should be checked, and the absorbent should be changed if needed. The circle and anesthetic machine should be tested for leaks. This is accomplished with the pop-off valve closed and the Y-piece occluded. The system is then filled with O_2, and the O_2 flow is set at 5 L/min. When the system pressure reaches 20 cmH$_2$O, the O_2 flow is gradually decreased until the pressure no longer rises. Any leak should be negligible.[2]

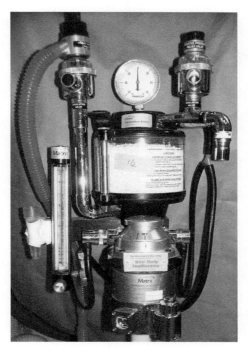

Figure 4.1   Anesthetic machine with a vaporizer.

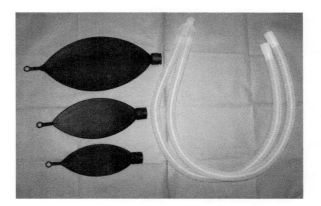

Figure 4.2   Rebreathing tubes and rebreathing bags.

There are two primary breathing systems used in veterinary medicine: rebreathing or "closed" and nonrebreathing or "semiclosed." The rebreathing system or circle system is referred to as a closed system because all or part of the expired gases is recirculated to the patient. This system is preferred for patients of average size and weight. The inspiratory and expiratory rebreathing tubes are connected by a Y-piece that is then connected to the endotracheal tube. The Universal F rebreathing circuit is a tube within a tube and can be used in place of the traditional Y-piece and breathing tubes[2] (Fig. 4.2). Pediatric rebreathing tubes should be used for animals weighing 10–15 lb (4.5–6.8 kg). A rebreathing bag is used to allow for the patient's tidal

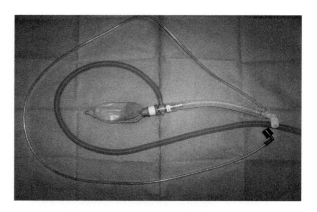

Figure 4.3   Bain nonrebreathing system.

volume and minimum volume during ventilation. The rebreathing bag should be 3–5 times the tidal volume (tidal volume is calculated at 10–15 mL/kg). The pop-off or adjustable pressure-limiting (APL) valve is an essential safety feature of a circle system. It vents excess gas and prevents the development of excessive pressure.[2] This valve should remain open at all times, except when manually ventilating the patient. A scavenger system is attached to the exit portal of the pop-off valve and eliminates waste gases from the environment. The nonrebreathing system is preferred for pediatric patients and those animals under 10 lb (4.5 kg). It induces less resistance to breathing and contains slightly less mechanical dead space than the circle system. Less inspiratory effort is required than with circle systems[2] (Fig. 4.3).

Before beginning the induction phase, all the necessary equipment should be prepared. Endotracheal tubes of various sizes should be available at the time of induction (see web content: "Anesthesia Cheat Sheet"). In general, three tubes are chosen: the size expected to be used, one size larger and one size smaller. The cuffs are inflated and checked for leaks before induction. The appropriate sized rebreathing tubes and rebreathing bag should be attached to the anesthetic machine. After intubation, the cuff is inflated only to the point where a seal will allow bagging at no more than 20 cmH$_2$O. An overinflated cuff can cause trauma to the delicate tissues of the trachea or even tracheal rupture. Once the patient is attached to the anesthetic machine, the oxygen flow rate and the anesthetic vaporizer settings are adjusted to maintenance levels. To achieve the correct amount of inflation of the endotracheal cuff, close the pop-off valve, then pressurize the system by squeezing the rebreathing bag. Add or remove air until you hear the gas leak at 15–20 cmH$_2$O. At this point, a patient can be maintained for a variable length of time. All monitoring equipment should be attached to the patient and baseline readings should be taken to begin the monitoring process (see web content: Video 4.1W Operatory Final).

Monitoring Anesthesia and Common Complications

Monitoring means the continued measurement of physiological variables over time.[3] Patients should be monitored during the entire anesthetic procedure up to and including part of the recovery phase. There are many multiparameter machines available (Fig. 4.4). Keep in mind that these machines should never be used as a substitute for

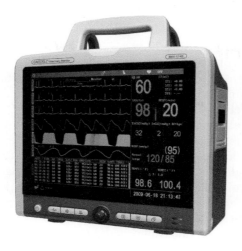

Figure 4.4   Multiparameter monitor (Courtesy of Jamie Renner, Midmark Animal Health).

hands-on human involvement in the monitoring process. An anesthetic record should be used for each patient, with values being recorded at least every 5–10 minutes until the patient is recovered from anesthesia. Once the procedure is completed, the anesthetic record should be placed in the patient's file and reviewed before the next anesthetic procedure. In addition to recording parameter data, the anesthetic record should also include the anesthetic protocol used for that particular patient. The anesthetic record essentially provides an accurate "picture" of how the patient is responding to the anesthesia. Any subtle changes from one reading to the next could indicate that the patient is either "too light" or "too deep" with regard to the anesthetic plane. This monitoring process also alerts the anesthetist of any abnormal vital signs, which can then be addressed early to avoid potential complications while the patient is under anesthesia. Preventing, as well as addressing complications, decreases the anesthetic risk and increases the chance for a favorable outcome.

Parameters that are most commonly monitored are oxygen saturation (pulse oximetry), respiration, ECG and heart rate, blood pressure, CO_2 levels (capnograph), and body temperature. Also, more invasive monitoring parameters may include blood gas analysis and central venous pressure.

Pulse Oximetry

Pulse oximetry measures the arterial oxyhemoglobin saturation of the patient. This allows the anesthetist to determine if the patient is receiving enough oxygen for healthy perfusion of organs and tissues. In most surgical patients, the probe is placed on the tongue. However, for dental patients, this can be cumbersome when working in the oral cavity. Alternative locations include the pinna, prepuce, vulva, toe, tail, or metacarpus. Oxygen saturation should be maintained between 98% and 100%, particularly if the animal is breathing 100% oxygen. Saturation readings of 90% or less indicate marked desaturation, hypovolemia, shock, or anemia.[4] It is important to determine the cause of desaturation to correct the problem. In many instances, the probe may have become dislodged after repositioning of the patient. Other causes can include low pressure in the oxygen supply or tank, low respirations, or poor ventilation of the patient.

Respiratory Monitor

Respiratory failure can lead directly to cardiovascular failure. For this reason, the respiratory rate is one of the most important parameters in the monitoring protocol. Apnea monitors are a crucial piece of equipment in alerting the anesthetist of increased, or more importantly, decreased respirations (Fig. 4.5). The monitor is placed between the rebreathing tubes and the endotracheal tube and emits an audible beep each time the animal takes a breath. An alarm of continuous beeping sounds when there is an excessive amount of time in between breaths. Changes in respiratory rate should be addressed to determine the cause. The increased respiratory rate could be due to a "light" anesthetic plane in which the animal is experiencing some degree of pain. A decreased respiratory rate could indicate a plane of anesthesia that is too "deep" and should be corrected. Apnea can occur immediately following induction. The patient should be given several breaths of oxygen immediately following induction. Breathing rates in normal dogs and cats vary between 10 and 50 breaths per minute, preoperatively or intraoperatively.[2]

ECG

Continuous monitoring of the ECG pattern allows early recognition of electrical changes associated with disorders of rate, rhythm, and conduction.[4] A decreased heart rate initially can be due to the premedications and induction but should stabilize once the procedure is started. Bradycardia requires definitive therapy when it causes an excessive decrease in cardiac output. An example would be when the heart rate decreases below 50–60 bpm in an animal that has an adequate circulating volume.[2] Sinus tachycardia (increased heart rate) is defined as a heart rate above 160 bpm in the dog and 180 bpm in the cat.[2] Causes of increased heart rate are underlying complications such as hypoxia, hypercapnia, or hyperthermia.

Blood Pressure

Hypotension is one of the most common complications of anesthesia. Unfortunately, blood pressure monitoring is often lacking in many veterinary practices. Blood pressure is influenced by the depth of anesthesia, blood volume, the strength of cardiac

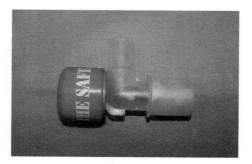

Figure 4.5 Apnea monitor.

contraction, systemic vascular resistance, and shock. The minimum mean arterial pressure (MAP) should not drop below 60 mmHg (systolic pressure below 80–90 mmHg) for vital organs to receive adequate perfusion.[3] Administering intravenous (IV) fluids throughout anesthesia may stabilize and maintain the blood pressure. Increasing the rate of administration of IV fluids and decreasing the depth of anesthesia may alleviate hypotension. Adding a colloid such as hetastarch and dopamine or dobutamine to the drip may be warranted in more severe or refractory hypotension.[5] The correct cuff size should be used to obtain accurate measurements. The cuff width should be 40% of the limb circumference in a dog and 30–40% in a cat.

Capnograph

Capnography measures the end-tidal CO_2 level in the anesthetic patient. End-tidal CO_2 is a graphic display of carbon dioxide pressure over time that allows assessment of ventilation, breathing circuit function, and ventilation–perfusion function in the lungs.[5] Respiratory responses to even subtle changes in CO_2 levels in the blood are extremely rapid because the chemoreceptors are much more sensitive to changes in CO_2 than to changes in O_2.[5] For this reason, capnography alerts the anesthetist much sooner to respiratory complications than pulse oximetry. Some common problems with ventilation can include improper placement of the endotracheal tube, partial or full obstruction, or apnea. The end-tidal CO_2 should be between 35 and 45 mmHg.[3]

Body Temperature

A dental procedure can last several minutes to several hours. Hypothermia can be a common occurrence with longer dental procedures, especially in cats and smaller breeds of dogs. Prolonged hypothermia can cause low respirations, bradycardia, decreased blood pressure, and a slow recovery. Consequently, these patients can become compromised without supportive care during the procedure or the recovery period. Unfortunately, maintaining body temperature is often overlooked and can be the cause of many unnecessary anesthetic deaths. The patient's body temperature should be monitored with a temperature probe or a simple thermometer, and controlled using a thermoregulatory system.

There are many options to choose from to maintain body temperature, including hot water blankets and heated air blankets (Fig. 4.6). The most effective method is one that is in contact or surrounds a good portion of the patient's body surface. A heated cage or incubator for smaller patients can be used as a recovery chamber to facilitate a smoother and shorter recovery period. Nonveterinary electric heating pads should be avoided as these may cause burn injuries to the patient. IV fluid line warmers are also available and are extremely helpful in maintaining the patient's body temperature.

Although unexplained or "fluke" reactions to anesthesia occur in a small percentage of cases, the majority of anesthetic emergencies arise from one or more of the following: inappropriate administration of anesthetic agents; poor monitoring or absence thereof; poor anesthetic equipment; lack of supportive therapy; or lack of timely intervention when complications do occur. Detecting complications early on and reacting quickly can increase the probability of a successful anesthetic event.

CHAPTER 4

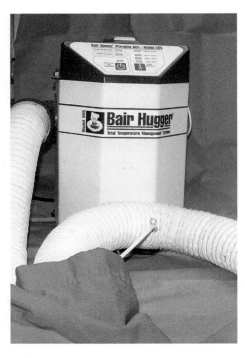

Figure 4.6   Heated air blanket heat source.

Pain Management in the Dental Patient

In veterinary dentistry, even noninvasive procedures can cause some degree of pain, with more invasive procedures being extremely painful. Although detrimental to any patient, pain is a particular problem for older patients with marginally compensated organ function. In patients with marginal cardiac, renal, or hepatic function, the stress of pain often results in decompensation during the procedure, during recovery, or in the days immediately after the procedure.[5] For this reason, effectively managing pain is vital to the patient's successful recovery. It is the role of the veterinary team to anticipate the needs of the patient and what type of pain relief the animal may need based on the procedure being performed. To be proficient in pain management, it is important first to understand how pain is received and transmitted.

Understanding the Pain Pathways

Pain is defined as a perception of noxious stimuli. Nociception is the processing of this noxious stimuli and perception of pain by the brain. Pain travels along three primary pathways before being perceived by the brain. In the dental patient, pain is introduced at the peripheral site, the oral cavity. This is known as transduction. After transduction, the painful stimulus is picked up by the peripheral nerves, which then carry it to the spinal cord. This is known as transmission. Finally, the spinal cord transfers the pain (a process known as modulation) to the brain, resulting in the perception of pain by the patient.[6] It is by interrupting the pain response along multiple pathways that the most effective pain management is achieved.

The Multimodal Approach to Pain

The use of two or more analgesics in combination to control pain is known as a multimodal approach to managing pain. This protocol is becoming widely recognized and utilized more frequently than in the past. There are a wide variety of parenteral analgesics that can be used to control pain along a specific pathway before, during, and after the dental procedure. Local anesthetics, nonsteroidal anti-inflammatory drugs (NSAIDs), opioids, and corticosteroids are used to control pain at the point of transduction. Local anesthetics and alpha-2 agonists are used at the point of transmission. Local anesthetics, opioids, and alpha-2 agonists are used with regard to modulation, and inhalant anesthetics at the point of perception. The timing of the use of these drugs is also a critical component of the pain management protocol.

Preemptive, as well as intraoperative and postoperative, pain management is the most efficacious. The goal of preemptive analgesia is to provide therapeutic intervention before a painful experience to prevent or minimize both peripheral and central nervous system (CNS) sensitization to the noxious stimulus.[6] Drugs that are given before the painful stimulus are much more effective than those same drugs administered after pain is introduced. By providing preemptive analgesia, postoperative pain is greatly reduced and much easier to control. This preemptive pain management begins with the premedicant sedation, usually an opioid or alpha-2 antagonist that interrupts pain at the site of modulation (spinal cord). For extremely painful dental procedures such as full-mouth extractions, mandibulectomy, or maxillectomy, a constant rate infusion started preoperatively and continued throughout and after the procedure can facilitate a smooth and pain-free recovery for the patient. A widely used combination for constant rate infusion includes an opioid (morphine) at a rate of 0.12–0.36 mg/kg/h, lidocaine at a rate of 0.6–1.5 mg/kg/h, and ketamine at a rate of 0.12–1.2 mg/kg/h.[7] Postoperatively, additional opioids and injectable NSAIDs can be administered to provide continued pain control following a procedure.

Regional Nerve Blocks

The regional nerve block is an extremely useful tool and should be part of the dental pain management arsenal. As part of the multimodal approach to pain control, the regional block stops the transmission of pain at the site of injury, preventing the painful stimulus from ever reaching the brain stem and, ultimately, the cerebral cortex. Local and regional anesthetics can enhance the effectiveness of the premedication and allows for a lower concentration of inhalant anesthetic needed to maintain a comfortable anesthetic plane. The block should be administered a few minutes before the painful procedure is begun for optimum effectiveness. Local or regional blocks are relatively simple to master with training and practice in a hands-on laboratory setting. Most technicians should be able to perform this task after completing a training program.

Regional blocks should be considered for many different oral procedures including extraction, root canal therapy, oral mass removal, maxillectomy, or mandibulectomy, and even for those advanced periodontal cases when aggressive open or closed root planing is performed. The drug of choice is usually lidocaine and bupivacaine, or bupivacaine alone. Each of these drugs has advantages and disadvantages.

Lidocaine has a short onset of action, but a very short duration lasting only 1–2 hours. Bupivacaine can last up to 6–10 hours but has a delayed onset of action. These limitations can be minimized or eliminated by using them in combination.[8] The total dose of bupivacaine should not exceed 2 mg/kg, with lidocaine not to exceed 5 mg/kg. The infused volume for each site is 0.25–1.0 mL depending on the size of the patient.[8] Lidocaine with epinephrine can be used as well to constrict blood vessels to aid in homeostasis but should be avoided in patients with underlying heart issues. A 25-gauge or 27-gauge needle on a 1 mL syringe is used to inject and deliver the drug into or near the foramen.

Infraorbital block

This foramen can be palpated through the buccal mucosa dorsal to the maxillary third premolar. This block provides analgesia from the maxillary third premolar to the incisors and the associated soft tissues. Holding the syringe parallel to the palate, the needle is inserted into the canal with the bevel up. The syringe is aspirated to avoid injecting into a blood vessel. The syringe is rotated until the bevel is facing down and aspiration is performed again before injecting slowly into the canal. Digital pressure is held over the site for 30–60 seconds to "hold" the drug in place to achieve the maximum effectiveness of the block.[8]

Maxillary nerve block

This block is also referred to as the caudal infraorbital nerve block. It affects the entire ipsilateral maxillary teeth and associated soft tissues. The foramen is located dorsal to the last maxillary molar. The needle is inserted vertically just caudal to the last molar with the bevel facing rostral or toward the nose of the patient. Aspiration is performed before injecting slowly near the foramen. Note that this nerve block has the potential to cause ocular trauma.[8]

Mandibular alveolar nerve block

The foramen is located on the lingual surface of the mandible, dorsal to the caudal ventral mandibular notch. This block provides analgesia to all the ipsilateral teeth and associated soft tissues and can be performed either intraorally or extraorally. Intraorally in the dog, the foramen is palpated on the lingual surface about halfway between the third molar and the angular process. In the cat, it is located halfway between the first molar and the angular process. Extraorally, the injection site is located on the lingual side of the mandible. The needle is inserted vertically at the mandibular notch on the lingual side of the mandible.[8]

Middle mental nerve block

There are three foramina located on the rostral portion of the mandible. The middle foramen is used as it is the largest of them. It is located ventral to the mesial root of the second premolar and affects all teeth and soft tissue rostral to the injection site. The needle is inserted parallel to the mandible at the base of the mandibular frenulum. The drug is delivered adjacent to the foramen. Digital pressure is applied for 30–60 seconds.

Local Nerve Block

A local nerve block provides analgesia only for a limited area. The drug is infused into the periodontal space or gingiva surrounding a tooth. This technique is used primarily for the extraction of incisors or for small oral mass removal. It is important to mention that these agents become ineffective when used in inflamed tissue due to changes in pH levels.[8]

Strategies for Home Pain Management

Once the patient is discharged, continued pain management is not only the best care for the patient, it also increases the possibility of owners consenting to future procedures if their pet is kept pain free at home. There is a myriad of home care strategies and drug protocols for dental patients. Choosing the correct protocol should be based on whether mild, moderate, or severe pain is anticipated based on the procedure performed. The physiological condition of the patient should also be taken into consideration. For moderate or severe pain, a multimodal approach should be employed. For example, an opioid given in conjunction with an NSAID can be a very effective combination. In dogs, the most common drugs used are meloxicam (0.2 mg/kg initially, then 0.1 mg/kg once daily) or carprofen (0.5 mg/kg twice daily), and tramadol (1–4 mg/kg two to three times daily). In cats, buprenorphine sublingually (0.1 mg/kg two to three times daily) is commonly used. In more severe cases, other drugs used may include gabapentin (3–5 mg/kg twice daily). This is used primarily in patients suffering from chronic or neuropathic pain, but it has been shown to provide effective analgesia in more severe dental cases. Liquid medications tend to be easier for an owner to administer than pills or capsules, especially if extensive dental work was performed. A reputable compounding pharmacy can be useful in formulating liquid medications when needed. The duration of administration of these drugs can vary, but most pain management protocols include a 5- to 7-day regimen of pain relief.

References

1. Peak, M. 2008. Marketing veterinary dentistry: creating value. Paper presented at the Florida Veterinary Medical Association Convention.
2. Hartsfield, S, Paddleford, R. 1999. *Manual of Small Animal Anesthesia*, 2nd edn (ed. R Paddleford). Philadelphia, PA: WB Saunders.
3. Stepaniuk, K, Brock, N. 2008. Anesthesia monitoring in the dental and oral surgery patient. *Journal of Veterinary Dentistry* 25:143–149.
4. Bellows, J. 2004. *Small Animal Dental Equipment, Materials and Techniques* (ed. N Albright). Ames, IA: Blackwell.
5. Holmstrom, S. 2000. *Veterinary Dentistry for the Technician and Office Staff* (ed. S Holmstrom). Philadelphia, PA: Elsevier Health Sciences.
6. Ko, J. 2008. New pain management techniques. *The NAVTA Journal* Spring:35–39.
7. Beckman, B. 2006. Pathophysiology and management of surgical and chronic pain in dogs and cats. *Journal of Veterinary Dentistry* 23:58.
8. Beckman, B. 2007. Regional nerve blocks key to delivering quality dental care. *DVM Newsmagazine*, September.

CHAPTER 4

The Dental Cleaning

5

Julie McMahon, LVT, VTS (Dentistry)

Learning Objectives

- Identify the instruments used to clean and polish teeth
- Describe the different types of dental records
- Identify the components of the dental record
- Perform the steps to prepare for the dental cleaning procedure before the patient is anesthetized
- Perform an oral exam with periodontal probing. Identify the abbreviations used for dental charting
- Chart oral exam findings on a dental record using dental terminology
- Perform a dental scaling using power instrumentation. Perform a dental scaling using hand instrumentation
- Perform the steps to polish teeth
- Perform a final examination of the oral cavity
- Describe the steps necessary to recover the dental patient. Identify home care products for dental patients
- Present a home care regimen for a dental patient
- Describe the steps required to perform instrument care. Describe the steps required to perform dental unit maintenance

Small Animal Dental Procedures for Veterinary Technicians and Nurses, Second Edition.
Edited by Jeanne R. Perrone.
© 2021 John Wiley & Sons, Inc. Published 2021 by John Wiley & Sons, Inc.

Introduction

Dental cleaning or prophylaxis is often only one step in a larger dental procedure. A dental prophylaxis is defined as a procedure that includes oral hygiene care, as well as techniques to prevent disease and remove plaque and calculus from the teeth above and beneath the gum line before periodontitis has occurred.[1] The goal is to aid in the prevention and control of gingival and periodontal infections and to create an environment where tissues can return to health. A prophylaxis may also be done in preparation for another dental procedure such as restorations, prosthodontics, orthodontics, and oral surgery.[2] A patient coming in for a prophylaxis often ends up needing periodontal therapy and/or oral surgery. Performing and assisting with dental procedures can be a rewarding aspect of a technician's career. We are able to be an active part of the procedure and make a difference in the animal's long-term health. The veterinary technician is often relied on to perform the prophylaxis and related tasks such as client education and going over home care instructions. The technician also aids in the documentation of oral pathology and acquires dental radiographs. This allows the veterinarian to form a treatment plan that is best for the patient.

Dental procedures should be done in a separate room. This is to reduce contamination of the rest of the hospital from bacterial aerosolization. You also need good lighting and ventilation. There are other ergonomic considerations. All equipment and instruments should be within reach. You should have good posture and be seated while working (Fig. 5.1).

Consider patient protection as well. Cuffed endotracheal tubes are a necessity to protect the patient from aerosolization and asphyxiation. A pharyngeal gauze pack may be used to minimize fluid pooling and minimize the risk of debris accumulating

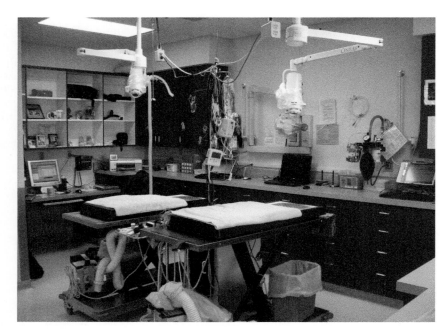

Figure 5.1　Dental procedures should be done in a separate room (Courtesy of John Koehm, DVM, FAVD).

around the endotracheal tube. If a pack is used, make sure that there is a tie attached to the pack to assure that you remember to remove it. The pack also needs to be changed frequently. Patients should be positioned for adequate drainage, with the head positioned lower in relation to the body. Although the oral cavity is not sterile, clean, sterile instruments should be used for each patient.

Common Instrumentation for the Dental Cleaning

There are various instruments used during the dental cleaning. In this section, we will cover the use of calculus removal forceps, power scalers, hand instruments, explorers, periodontal probes, and polishing instruments. Power instruments, such as sonic and ultrasonic scalers, use rapid energy vibrations to fracture calculus from a tooth surface and to clean periodontal pockets as needed.[3] Hand instruments are used for fine-tuning after power scaling.

Calculus Removal Forceps

Calculus removal forceps are used for removal of large deposits of calculus from the tooth surface at the beginning of a procedure.[4] This is a very powerful instrument and should be used with great care as you can inadvertently damage a tooth or surrounding soft tissues. The forceps are similar in design to extraction forceps except that one side of the working end has a straight tip and the other has a curved tip to help engage the margin of the calculus near the gingival margin. To use the forceps, grasp the handle and place the straight end on the palatal/lingual surface of the tooth and the curved on the buccal surface at the margin of the calculus just below the gingiva. Gently squeeze the handle and pull down at the crown of the tooth. This will remove the very large thick pieces of calculus. It should not be used to remove smaller pieces.

Power Instruments

Sonic scalers are driven by compressed air, and the tip oscillates at a sonic frequency. Ultrasonic scalers are more commonly used and are driven by a micromotor with a tip that oscillates at an ultrasonic frequency. Each scaler operates differently and has various tips and inserts to perform scaling (Fig. 5.2). (See Chapter 3 for further details.)

Rotary scalers are best avoided because they are known to cause pain and significant enamel damage. Rotoburs fit in a high-speed handpiece to remove the calculus. This is considered an obsolete method of calculus removal and is not recommended.

Instruments for the Oral Exam

When performing an oral exam, there are a few instruments needed. This includes a periodontal probe, explorer, and a dental mirror (see Video 7.1W Periodontal hand instrumentation).

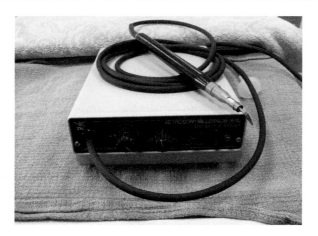

Figure 5.2   Ultrasonic dental scaler (Courtesy of John Koehm, DVM, FAVD).

Periodontal probe

Periodontal probes are used to measure the gingival sulcus, as well as periodontal pocket depth; determine gingival inflammation, furcation exposure, and tooth mobility; and measure the size of oral lesions. They are round or flat instruments with a graduated blunt end used for measurement. They come in various lengths with millimeters marked on them.[5] Examples are round (#14 Williams B) and flat (Goldman-Fox).

Dental explorer

The explorer is a sharp-ended instrument that is straight or curved. It is used to check for caries, enamel or dentin defects, fractures, tooth resorption, and subgingival calculus. Examples are a straight #6 and the more common shepherd's hook. They commonly come double ended with an explorer on one end and a periodontal probe on the other.

Dental mirror

Dental mirrors are used to better visualize palatal, lingual, and distal molar surfaces. They also reflect light onto surfaces and retract soft tissue. There are small and large circular mirrors.

Dental polishing

Dental polishing removes plaque and smooths enamel surfaces after scaling. It is done with a low-speed handpiece, a prophy angle, prophy cup, and polish. Air polishing is similar to sandblasting. It uses bicarbonate of soda, and you must protect oral tissues because it can cause significant damage.[6]

Instruments for the Dental Cleaning

There are two main types of hand instruments needed for the dental cleaning. First is the scaler, which is used for supragingival scaling. Second is the curette, which is used for both supra- and subgingival scaling. Both scalers and curettes require frequent sharpening.

Hand scalers

Hand scalers are for supragingival scaling only.[7] In general, scalers are sturdier and should be used more for general calculus removal than a curette. The cross-section of a scaler is triangular and has two cutting edges. The sharp working tip can cause trauma to the gingiva. Common types of dental scalers are the sickle scaler (curved) and the Jacquette scaler (straight).

Hand curettes

Hand curettes are primarily for the removal of subgingival calculus, but they can also be used supragingivally. They are more slender than a scaler and have a rounded back and tip.

Curettes can be used supra- and subgingivally; however, they are considered to be more delicate than a scaler and should not be used as one. This usage will age your instrument quickly. The curette has a rounded tip or toe, and its cross-section is a half-moon shape. This design is more forgiving on the gingival tissues. There are two main types. First is the universal curette, which can be used almost anywhere in the mouth. Second is the Gracey curette, which has only one cutting edge and is area specific (Fig. 5.3).

Power equipment

A micromotor is used for polishing and can be used for tooth sectioning for extraction. The main problem is the absence of water, which requires an external source, to prevent thermal damage. Some micromotors do not have high enough revolutions per minute (rpm) for sectioning. Compressed air units have a high-speed handpiece with water coolant, a low-speed handpiece without water, and air/water syringe. These can have satellite compressors or be all in one. This is ideal for everyday use. (See Chapter 3 for further details.)

The Dental Record

As part of the patient's complete record, the dental record is a legal document and is an essential part of a dental procedure. It is utilized to document information about the patient, pathology, and procedure. These records can be in many different forms but all should include the following information with the anatomical chart: the client information, patient information, complaint, medical history, dental history, exam findings, radiographic interpretation, treatment plan, consent for treatment, documentation of treatment, prognosis, and follow-up care recommendations. There should also be documentation of client discussions and consultations with other professionals. There are several different types and styles of dental charts available for you to choose from, including stickers, paper, and computerized charts. The record may be a single page or several pages depending on the use of other documents, such as patient release forms, separate anesthesia monitoring sheets, or other documents that might complement the dental record.

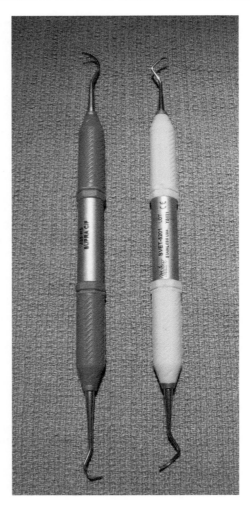

Figure 5.3 Hand scalers (left) are for supragingival scaling only. Curettes (right) are for the removal of subgingival calculus as well as supragingival calculus (Courtesy of John Koehm, DVM, FAVD).

Dental stickers are good when combined with the patient's records; however, they are self-limiting because of their size, which makes it difficult to fit the pathology, plan, treatment, or other documentation in the available space. Depending on the style of the label, the teeth will be laid out with either a buccal, occlusal, and lingual view or just an open-mouth occlusal view.

Paper charts are typically printed on a full 8.5 × 11-inch (216 × 279 mm) sheet of paper with room on the front and back for complete documentation of the procedure. The front of the document allows for the overall exam of the head and oral cavity, including facial symmetry, swellings, occlusal evaluation, skull type, and soft tissue exam. You can also document overall plaque, calculus, gingivitis, and other tooth abnormalities. The back includes an anatomical chart with buccal, occlusal, and lingual views for charting. There is also space for your plan, treatments performed, and additional notes.

Computerized charts are newer and in many systems are a work in progress. There are tablet systems that display the chart and allow for editing with a pen or insertion of text. It then can be saved as a document attached to the patient's record. This allows for the diversity of a paper chart with computerized storage in a paperless setting. It also allows for the patient's information to be imported to the chart from your management software. It will enable drawings and shapes to be inserted in different colors to more clearly document pathology. Additional notes and images can be added as well. Other systems have charts that are attached to practice management software. These also allow for drawing and shape placement for charting but do not allow the freedom and ease of charting that a paper chart or tablet does. (See Appendices 2 and 3 for sample canine and feline dental charts.)

When charting the mouth, a combination of abbreviations, marks, drawings, and written explanations are used to thoroughly document the pathology. There are a myriad of abbreviations and terminology that are available to aid in charting. Much of the anatomical and directional terminology that is necessary for charting is covered in Chapter 1. A current and complete list of abbreviations can be found at the American Veterinary Dental College website (https://avdc.org/wp-content/uploads/2019/08/abbreviations.pdf). Table 5.1 presents a list of abbreviations commonly used by technicians.[8]

Tooth identification on the dental chart can be done in one of two ways: the anatomical system or the modified Triadan system.[9]

Anatomical System

The anatomical system uses a combination of letters and numbers to identify each tooth (I = incisor; C = canine; PM = premolar; M = molar). A number is placed around the letter to indicate which tooth it is, as well as the location. (e.g., I^1 = right upper first incisor; ^3PM = left upper third premolar). Deciduous teeth are notated by lowercase letters. This system is easy to learn; however, it is more time-consuming and difficult to use with most computerized systems.

Triadan System

The Triadan system is a numbering system that uses three numbers to identify each tooth. The first number indicates the quadrant the tooth is in (100 = right maxilla; 200 = left maxilla; 300 = left mandible; 400 = right mandible). The next two numbers indicate the tooth, beginning from the midline out. The central incisor is 01, the middle incisor is 02, the lateral incisor is 03, the canine is 04, premolar 1 is 05, and molar 1 is 09. The three numbers then tell exactly which tooth you are identifying (e.g., 204 = left maxillary canine; 409 = right mandibular first molar). There is a rule of 4 and 9 that states that a canine is always 04 and a first molar is always 09. This is helpful when working with animals that are missing teeth or have supernumerary teeth. Deciduous teeth are indicated by adding 400 to the quadrant the tooth is in. If the deciduous tooth is in the 100 quadrant, it would be a 500; if the tooth is in the 400 quadrant, it would be an 800 (e.g., 604 = left maxillary deciduous canine; 706 = left mandibular deciduous second premolar).[9] The Triadan system is being used more in practice because of the ease of use with a computerized system (Fig. 5.4).

Table 5.1   Common abbreviations used by veterinary technicians

Diagnostic		Diagnostic	
AB	Abrasion	SN	Supernumerary tooth
AT	Attrition	T/FX	Tooth fracture
C	Canine	TR(1–5)	Tooth resorption
CA	Caries		
CI(0–3)	Calculus index	**Treatment**	
E	Enamel		
E/D	Enamel defect	B/I	Biopsy incisional
F(1–3)	Furcation exposure	B/E	Biopsy excisional
FX	Fracture	FX/R	Fracture repair
GE	Gingival enlargement (no histopathology)	GTR	Guided tissue regeneration
GH	Gingival hyperplasia	GV	Gingivectomy
GI	Gingivitis index	PRO	Prophylaxis
GR	Gingival recession	R	Restoration
MAL	Malocclusion	RAD	Radiograph
M(1–3)	Mobility	RC	Root canal therapy
ONF	Oronasal fistula	RPC	Root plane closed
PD(0–4)	Periodontal disease (0–4)	RPO	Root plane open
PI(0–3)*	Plaque index (0–3)	S	Surgery
PE	Pulp exposure	X	Simple extraction (closed no sectioning)
PM or P	Premolar	XS	Extraction with sectioning of tooth (closed sectioning)
Rad	Radiograph		
RD	Retained deciduous tooth	XSS	Surgical extraction (open and sectioning)
RTR	Retained root		

Setting Up a Charting Protocol

When charting, it is important to use a specific repetitive pattern to make sure you do not miss a quadrant. One method is to work with the patient in lateral recumbency; the work is done on one side, then the patient is rolled over, and the procedure is

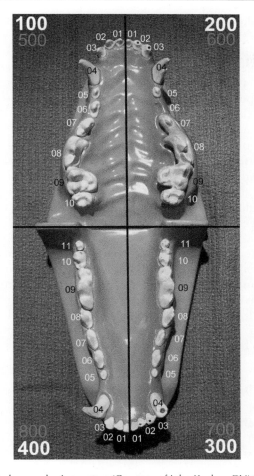

Figure 5.4   Modified Triadan numbering system (Courtesy of John Koehm, DVM, FAVD).

repeated. When charting with this method, you will document the buccal sides of the top (up) teeth and the palatal/lingual sides of the bottom (down) teeth. The exact pattern that you use does not matter as long as you cover all surfaces of the teeth and you keep using the same pattern. An example would be to start at the maxillary midline and work your way distally on the buccal side, and then do the same with the mandible. Next, look at the palatal surface of the opposing side, starting at the midline and move distally; repeat this process on the lingual portion of the mandibular teeth.

The Dental Cleaning Procedure

Preparation

Part of the preparation for a cleaning is making sure the client is aware of all aspects of the procedure and has signed the appropriate paperwork. This includes, but is not limited to, cost, anesthesia and associated risks, steps of the procedure, recovery, home care, and follow-up. (See Chapter 2 for further details.)

All patients should have an intravenous catheter placed and have a balanced electrolyte solution run during anesthesia. Consider the patient's preanesthetic medications based on their history, health, and American Society of Anesthesiologists Physical Status Scale. This often includes antibiotics, preanesthetic sedation, and pain management, as well as induction and maintenance anesthetic agents, and intraoperative and postoperative medications. The use of a cuffed endotracheal tube is necessary for the delivery of anesthesia as well as to protect the patient from aspiration of debris. (See Chapter 4 for further details.)

The preparation of your work area is the key to the ease of your procedure. This will assure the shortest anesthetic event for the patient. Prepare your dental chart and anesthetic monitoring sheet. Pressure-check your anesthetic machine and be sure to have the correct size of tubing and bag. Your monitoring equipment, fluids, and infusion pump should also be ready. Prepare your dental unit, which will include the high-speed handpiece, low-speed handpiece, air/water syringe, and power scaler. Other instruments will consist of a power scaler inserts/tips, various hand scalers and curettes, a periodontal probe, dental explorer, prophy angle, prophy cup, and paste. Other materials needed include a dental mirror, calculus removal forceps, a mouth speculum, and gauze for a pharyngeal pack. A chlorhexidine solution for flushing the oral cavity before the procedure will reduce bacterial aerosolization.[10] Have your personal protection equipment ready, which should include a minimum of a mask, eye protection, and gloves. Good lighting and magnification are invaluable and should also be available (see Chapter 3).

Purpose of the Oral Exam and Charting

The oral exam and charting is one of the most important steps in a dental procedure. The technician often performs this along with the prophylaxis. The oral exam should be done in a systematic, organized manner much like when performing the cleaning.[3] In order to successfully identify oral pathology, you must know what the normal anatomy is. The documentation of the oral exam on a dental record then becomes part of the patient's complete record. As stated before, the dental record is a legal document and is an essential part of a dental procedure.

The oral exam

The patient's oral exam is intended to determine if there is any presence of disease and if so, the type, extent, and severity. Always consider the whole patient: signs and symptoms, medical history, medications, and behavior during the process.[11] The oral exam begins in the exam room with the awake patient and the client. This part of the exam is covered in detail in Chapter 2. Some of the awake and anesthetized exams can overlap, although it is better to duplicate than miss any pathology. Some of the exams can also be done while the patient is sedated prior to anesthesia. This will include documentation of the skull type and any abnormalities with facial symmetry, swellings of the face, lymph nodes, and salivary glands. You may also be able to document the occlusion and count the teeth.

Once the patient is anesthetized and before the endotracheal tube is placed, the oropharynx region should be examined.[12] This will include the tonsils and their crypts, soft palate, fauces, uvula, and the palatoglossal arch. When examining these areas, look for redness, swelling, ulcers, oral masses, trauma, tonsillitis, and foreign bodies.

After placing the endotracheal tube, continue your soft tissue exam with the hard palate. Examine the rugae fold symmetry and look for other defects. Check all of these areas for redness, swelling, ulcers, masses, trauma, and foreign bodies. Next, examine the cheeks, lips, and commissures for fold pyoderma, masses, and possible signs of autoimmune disease. Continue with the tongue and floor of the mouth, looking for mobility, ulcers, foreign bodies, masses, swellings, or the presence of a ranula. Examine the mucosa and gingiva for color, redness, texture, swelling, moisture, discharge, fistula, ulcers, kissing lesions, masses, and wounds. The gingiva should also be examined for hyperplasia, recession, and other signs related to periodontal disease. Find the salivary papilla and look for inflammation. The papilla is located above the maxillary fourth premolar, sublingually. In the cat, there is one located just lingual to the mandibular first molar[13] (Fig. 5.5).

Periodontal exam

The periodontal exam helps determine if there is a presence of periodontal disease.[12] Make sure you are being systematic with your exam and starting at the same point each time while documenting all abnormalities. Materials needed for a periodontal exam are a dental mirror, a periodontal probe, and a dental explorer. When performing a periodontal exam, there are a number of different indicators to identify periodontal disease. This includes the following: plaque index, calculus index, gingivitis index, periodontal pocket depth, gingival hyperplasia, root exposure, tooth mobility, furcation exposure, total attachment loss, and any other oral lesions noted.

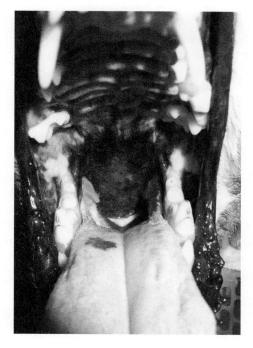

Figure 5.5 Once the patient is anesthetized and before the endotracheal tube is placed, the oropharynx region should be examined (Courtesy of John Koehm, DVM, FAVD).

Charting Your Findings

Plaque and calculus are evaluated by a visual exam. The plaque index and calculus index are quantitative measurements that allow you to document the presence of plaque and calculus. It is advised that you record the amount of plaque or calculus per tooth versus as a whole because it can help you determine patterns of disease. For example, if a dog is in pain and favoring the left side, you are likely to see more plaque and calculus on that side. When an area is not being used, it will build more plaque and calculus, likely causing more gingivitis and opportunities for periodontal disease. This means that you need to pay extra attention to areas with more buildup (see web content: Presentation 7.1W Stages of periodontal disease).

Plaque index (PI0–3)

The plaque index is a measurement of plaque detected on the surface of each tooth. A plaque index of 0 (PI0) means that there is no visible plaque on the surface. A plaque index of 1 (PI1) means that there is plaque covering less than one-third of the surface. A plaque index of 2 (PI2) means that there is plaque covering between one-third and two-thirds of the tooth surface. A plaque index of 3 (PI3) means that there is plaque covering more than two-thirds of the tooth surface.[14]

Calculus index (CI0–3)

The calculus index is a measurement of calculus detected on the surface of each tooth. A calculus index of 0 (CI0) means that there is no visible calculus on the surface. A calculus index of 1 (CI1) means that there is calculus covering less than one-third of the surface. A calculus index of 2 (CI2) means that there is calculus covering between one-third and two-thirds of the tooth surface with minimal subgingival involvement. A calculus index of 3 (CI3) means that there is calculus covering more than two-thirds of the tooth surface, with significant subgingival involvement.[14]

Gingivitis index (GI0–3)

Gingivitis is evaluated by a combination of visual inspections and the use of a periodontal probe. When visually examining the gingiva, you are looking for the presence of redness and inflammation. The probe is used to gently touch the gingiva at the gingival margin of each tooth to determine if any bleeding is present. The gingivitis index is a measurement of the gingivitis detected. It is advised that you document gingivitis on each tooth versus as a whole because it can also indicate patterns of disease.

A gingivitis index of 0 (GI0) means that there is no gingival inflammation. A gingivitis index of 1 (GI1) means that there is inflammation but no bleeding upon probing. A gingivitis index of 2 (GI2) means that there is moderate inflammation and bleeding upon probing. A gingivitis index of 3 (GI3) means that there is severe inflammation and spontaneous bleeding will be present.[14]

Counting the teeth

Counting the teeth should be one of the first steps in your exam. When you are counting teeth, you are looking for extra (supernumerary) teeth and missing teeth. Supernumerary teeth are commonly incisors and first premolars; however, they can be any tooth. When evaluating these teeth, consider whether or not they are causing any problems. Many supernumerary teeth do not cause a problem and can simply be documented and left alone. If a supernumerary tooth is causing crowding that will allow periodontal disease to occur, then extraction of the tooth should be considered. Supernumerary teeth should be drawn onto the chart. Missing teeth occur quite frequently. Common teeth to be missing are the maxillary and mandibular first premolars (105, 205, 305, and 405) and mandibular third molars (311, 411), although any tooth can be missing. When encountering a missing tooth, it should be radiographed. This is to help determine if the tooth is truly missing, impacted, or if there is the presence of retained roots. If a tooth is truly missing, then there is no need for any further treatment. A missing tooth is circled on the dental chart and abbreviated with an "O."

Impacted teeth are teeth that are still under the gingiva and bone. If not detected early, these can result in dentigerous cyst formation and can lead to significant bone loss and tooth destruction. In some cases, these can lead to neoplasia formation. Impacted teeth are abbreviated as T/I.

Retained roots are the result of the loss of crown. This can occur from fractures, tooth resorption, or from a previous unsuccessful attempt to extract a tooth. Retained roots can also cause long-term infections and should be evaluated and removed when appropriate. Retained roots are abbreviated as RTR.

Periodontal probing

When evaluating periodontal pocketing around a tooth, you should check each tooth in four to six places with your periodontal probe with a gentle walking stroke. A walking stroke is a series of bobbing strokes along the junctional epithelium with forward movements in 1 mm increments while moving the probe 1–2 mm up and down. When performing the probing, the tip of the probe (1–2 mm) should maintain contact with the tooth while keeping it parallel to the long axis of the tooth.[3] After cleaning one side of the mouth, probe the buccal surfaces of the maxillary teeth and the lingual surfaces of the mandibular teeth. Repeat the probing procedure on the other side. The normal gingival sulcus depth is 0–3 mm for dogs and 0–1 mm for cats. Measurements greater than this are considered to be a sign of periodontal disease and need to be documented on the dental chart. A periodontal pocket is an indicator of periodontal ligament attachment loss and bone loss.[12]

It is important to take into consideration the size of the patient when probing. A Yorkie with a 3 mm pocket is likely to have periodontal disease, whereas a Great Dane may have a 5 mm pocket on a canine and it may be normal for that dog. Some patients may have inflammation or gingival enlargement, which will create artificial probing depths. These are known as pseudopockets and do not truly reflect the loss of attachment of the periodontal ligament or bone.[15]

Gingival enlargement is the growth of excess gingival tissues and is measured in millimeters from the top of the gingival margin to the sulcus. You may also see gingival enlargement and a periodontal pocket at the same time, so there may be a measurement of the enlargement as well as the pocket.

Gingival recession, root exposure, and attachment loss

Root exposure occurs when gingival recession and bone loss occurs around a tooth. It is measured in millimeters from the cementoenamel junction of the tooth to the

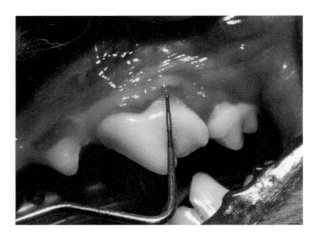

Figure 5.6   Total attachment loss is the combined total of periodontal pocketing and root exposure (Courtesy of John Koehm, DVM, FAVD).

gingival margin. Total attachment loss is the combined total of periodontal pocketing and root exposure (Fig. 5.6).

Tooth mobility (M1–3)

Tooth mobility is measured by how much a tooth moves from its axis in millimeters. Using a periodontal probe, engage the tooth, rocking it back and forth horizontally. Some teeth have mobility that is considered normal for them. An example would be the mandibular incisors. Mobility of stage 0 (M0) is a normal physiological movement up to 0.2 mm. Mobility of stage 1 (M1) is increased movement in any direction other than axial of 0.2 mm and up to 0.5 mm. Mobility of stage 2 (M2) indicates increased movement in any direction other than axial of 0.5 mm and up to 1.0 mm. With mobility of stage 3 (M3), the movement is increased in any direction of more than 1.0 mm.[16]

Furcation exposure (F1–3)

The furcation is the area where the roots of multirooted teeth come together. In a healthy mouth, the furcations are not visible or significantly palpable on exam. Furcation exposure is a result of periodontal disease, causing gingival recession and bone loss around the teeth. Furcation exposures are measured by grades 1–3. A furcation exposure of grade 1 (F1) exists when a periodontal probe extends less than halfway under the crown in any direction of a multirooted tooth with attachment loss. On exam, the periodontal probe will fall into the depression but bounce back out with little or no resistance. A furcation exposure of grade 2 (F2) exists when a periodontal probe extends greater than halfway under the crown of a multirooted tooth with attachment loss but not through and through. On exam, the periodontal probe will fall into the depression and readily stay. A furcation exposure of grade 3 (F3) exists when a periodontal probe extends under the crown of a multirooted tooth and passes from one side of the furcation to the other.[17]

When determining how to treat furcation exposures, the veterinarian will need to evaluate several factors. This will include the client's willingness to perform daily home care and the health of the surrounding teeth. Furcation exposures of 1 and 2 may not need to be extracted if they can be maintained with proper home care and regular professional visits. However, because periodontal disease is considered to be progressive, they often need eventual extraction if follow-up treatment is not provided. Grade 3 furcation exposures are usually extracted to prevent the advancement of periodontal disease to the tooth and surrounding teeth.

Retained/persistent deciduous teeth

Retained/persistent deciduous teeth frequently occur on small-breed dogs but can occur with any dog or cat. Deciduous canines (504, 604, 704, 804) are the most common tooth to be retained. Retained deciduous teeth can cause occlusion problems as well as an increase in the incidence of periodontal disease. Retained deciduous teeth should be radiographed to make sure there is a succedaneous tooth and to evaluate the root structure before extracting. If there is a deciduous tooth that has no successor, some believe that it may be left in and evaluated at a later date, as a deciduous tooth is better than no tooth. Retained deciduous teeth are drawn in on the chart and abbreviated as RD.

Wear: abrasion versus attrition

Wear is a more common occurrence in a dog's mouth than in a cat's and is characterized as the loss of enamel and dentin from repeated friction on the teeth.[18] There are two types of wear: abrasion and attrition.

Abrasion is wear that results from an external source, such as tennis balls, Frisbees, cage chewing, and dermatitis wear. The patterns are very distinct on examination. Wear patterns from tennis balls have a concave pattern on the occlusal surfaces of the maxillary and mandibular teeth, starting at the canines and running distally to the upper fourth premolars. Heavy play with Frisbees can cause a flat wear pattern on the incisors and canines. Cage chewers have wear on the distal surfaces of the canines, incisors, and occasionally on the premolars. If this behavior continues, the teeth can fracture, causing pulp exposure. Dogs with pruritic skin conditions can have wear due to chewing on their fur and skin for long periods of time. This abrasion is on the canines and incisors and can be flat or angled rostrally. Abrasion is drawn on the teeth that are affected and abbreviated as AB.

Attrition is the result of tooth-to-tooth contact. It is also referred to as occlusal wear.[19] Attrition is often a result of a malocclusion, causing teeth to have abnormal contact with each other. Examples are with animals with a Class 3 malocclusion where the mandibular canines come in contact with the maxillary third incisors. Over time, the canines and the incisors wear down, causing loss of tooth structure. Attrition is drawn on the chart and abbreviated as AT.

If wear occurs slowly over a long period of time, the body can keep pace and continue to lay down reparative dentin, allowing the pulp to recede and remain protected. This appears on the tooth as a reddish-brown stain and feels very smooth when an explorer is run perpendicularly over the worn area.[13] If the wear occurs faster than the tooth can keep up, then pulp exposure can occur. All teeth with wear should be radiographed to evaluate the vitality of the tooth.

Malformed teeth

When examining the teeth, look for malformations. This again goes back to knowing what normal looks like. Malformations may be seen in the crowns, developmental groove, and on the roots of the teeth and are often the result of trauma during development. When detected, these findings should be drawn in, and a written description should accompany it.

Malpositioned teeth

Malpositioned teeth can be crowded and/or rotated. Crowded and rotated teeth frequently occur with brachycephalic breeds. They are also seen when there are supernumerary teeth present. When evaluating these teeth, look for areas where periodontal disease can potentially arise. Crowded teeth are abbreviated as CWD, and rotated teeth are abbreviated as ROT, with an arrow drawn over the tooth indicating the direction of the rotation.

Enamel hypoplasia/hypocalcification

Enamel hypoplasia is a loss of enamel on the tooth surface. This can be the result of trauma to the developing tooth bud or when fever occurs during tooth development. Enamel hypoplasia can be located on one tooth or can be generalized throughout the mouth. Enamel hypoplasia is abbreviated as E/H and should be drawn in on the chart.

Trauma

Tooth trauma can result in several problems. Anterior teeth are often damaged by blunt force. Catching Frisbees, fetching rocks, running into stationary objects, tug of war, and cage chewing are examples of events that can cause injuries. Posterior teeth are usually injured by chewing aggressively on objects such as bones, hooves, hard nylon bones, wood, and rocks. When the injury occurs, it can result in fracture, pulpal hemorrhage, disruption of the apical blood supply, and in some cases luxation (partial displacement of the tooth from the socket) or avulsion (complete displacement of the tooth from the socket).

Tooth fractures are classified based on the degree of the fracture. Fractures are abbreviated as T/FX/(type of fracture).

Pulpal hemorrhage is when bleeding has occurred within the pulp canal, causing increased pressure on the nerves and blood supply. This often results in the death of the tooth. The exception to this is if the trauma occurs to a young animal. Because there is a large pulp chamber, there is room for expansion of the inflamed tissue, giving the tooth a chance to survive. Pulpal hemorrhage causes a discoloration of the injured tooth. An early injury will have a pinkish-purple color, and as the hemoglobin decomposes the color changes to a tan-brown. The abbreviation for this is T/NV.

Complete disruption of the apical blood supply will result in the death of the tooth. This can be a luxation or an avulsion and is usually due to a traumatic injury. A luxation will present with the patient having a tooth that is loose in the socket and may have obvious areas of torn gingiva and fractured alveolar bone. A luxated tooth is abbreviated as T/LUX. With avulsions, the patient is presented with the tooth out of the socket, and they also may have obvious torn gingiva and alveolar bone fractures. An avulsed tooth is abbreviated as T/A.

Tooth resorption

Tooth resorption can occur in both dogs and cats. It is a process by which all or part of a tooth structure is lost due to the destruction of mineralized tissue, mediated by odontoclasts.[19] This includes cementum, dentin, and enamel. Tooth resorption is detected by visual inspection of the gingiva for "band-aid lesions." These are patches of granulation tissue that are found on the crown of a diseased tooth covering the lesion caused by the resorption. Tooth resorption can also be detected with an explorer by running it perpendicular to the tooth at the gingival margin. If a lesion is present, the explorer will catch at the margin of the defect. Dental radiographs are also necessary for the detection and classification of tooth resorption.

Tooth resorption is classified into five stages, with several substages within. It is abbreviated as TR followed by the stage number the tooth is in. (See Chapter 8 for details on tooth resorption and its classifications.)

Caries

True dental caries are uncommon in dogs and almost unheard of in cats. Caries are characterized as demineralization of the hard dental tissues from acids created in plaque. The acids are formed from the oral bacteria fermenting carbohydrates, converting them into acids.[20] Caries usually present as small black lesions on the enamel in early stages. If caries have started to develop, you will be able to force the tip of the explorer into the decaying surface. As you withdraw the instrument, the tip will stick and let go, resulting in a metallic ping from the explorer tip.[21] Advanced caries often result in substantial tooth loss and pulp exposure. Caries are abbreviated as CA and drawn on the chart (see web content: Skillbuilder for Basics of the Dental Cleaning and Video 5.1W Basics of the Dental Cleaning Part 1).

Cleaning the Teeth Using the Power Scaler

When working with power scalers, it is important to know the machine you are using because each one has its own specifications on how to use it properly. This is especially true when it comes to water and power settings in relation to the type of tips that are being used. Find your user's manual and read it before using your machine.

An indication for the use of the power scaler is the buildup of calculus on the tooth surface. Scalers are used along with calculus removal forceps to quickly remove large deposits of calculus and clean the surface of the tooth. When indicated, power scaling is also used to remove subgingival calculus, plaque, and associated diseased tissues. This can include necrotic soft tissues and cementum.

When working with a power scaler, it is important to use proper technique (Fig. 5.7). A light grasp should be used when holding the instrument. Someone should be able to come up behind you and pull the handpiece out of your hand without resistance when you are scaling. In order for the instrument to work correctly, it should be balanced in your hand with little pull from the cord.[6] The modified pen grasp is not necessary; however, the use of a fulcrum is helpful. You can also loop the cord around a finger to reduce the pull on your hand.

Water serves a dual purpose in power scaling. First, the proper amount of water is vital during the use of the scaler because it decreases the heat generated by the

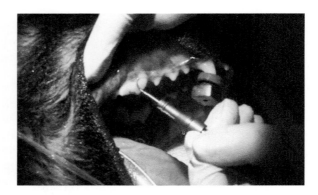

Figure 5.7   Power scaling is used to remove subgingival calculus, plaque, and associated diseased tissues (Courtesy of John Koehm, DVM, FAVD).

scaler. In general, the larger the tip, the more water needed; the smaller the tip, the less water needed. The second purpose is cavitation. Cavitation occurs when the water exits the tip of the instrument as a mist. Within the mist are tiny bubbles that collapse, releasing energy that serves to flush away calculus, plaque, and debris as well as destroy bacteria through tearing of the cell walls.[3,11]

The proper power setting is also very important. Most supragingival tips can be run at a medium to high power setting. Subgingival tips are run at low to medium power settings. A new tip is going to require less power, but as it ages the metal tip wears down, and a gradual increase of power may be needed. Never use a subgingival tip higher than a medium power setting as it can damage the instrument as well as the tooth. If after increasing the power the tip is unable to clean the tooth surface effectively, it should be replaced right away.

Light pressure should be used when engaging the tip to the tooth. Too much pressure creates excessive heat and hinders the vibrations of the scaler, which prevents it from working efficiently. This also causes unnecessary etching on the tooth surface. On the reverse, your pressure should not be too light because you will not engage the calculus and your instrument will be ineffective. It is ideal to use the back and lateral surfaces of the tip, keeping it parallel to the tooth's long axis and moving with a combination of short, overlapping, vertical, oblique, and horizontal strokes.[3] When working on a tooth surface, keep moving and do not spend more than 10–15 seconds on each tooth. If too much heat is a concern, you can cool the tooth with water between scaling. Depending on the type of tip and machine, there will be anywhere from 3 to 12 mm of active surface to work with. In general, the most terminal 4 mm of the tip are the most useful for calculus removal. Do not use the tip or face of the instrument because they are the most active surfaces and can cause damage to the tooth surface.[3]

The use of power scalers is contraindicated when restorations are present. Sonic and ultrasonic instruments can cause restorations to become dislodged. Gently clean areas with restorations with hand instruments as an alternative.

Dental Cleaning with Hand Instrumentation

Hand instrumentation was used exclusively in veterinary dentistry before power scalers. Today, it is performed in conjunction with power scaling. Hand

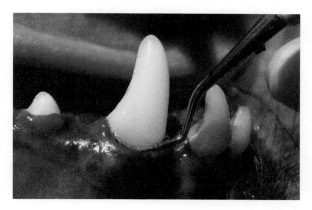

Figure 5.8 Hand instrumentation is the use of scalers and curettes to fine-tune the cleaning after power scaling (Courtesy of John Koehm, DVM, FAVD).

instrumentation is the use of scalers and curettes to fine-tune the cleaning after power scaling (Fig. 5.8). Power scaling cannot remove all calculus or plaque; therefore, no dental cleaning is complete with just power scaling. The leftover calculus will allow for new plaque and calculus to build up quickly.

Common areas that residual calculus is found are on the upper fourth premolars and both upper molars, as well as the lingual surfaces of the mandibular premolars. To detect any remaining calculus, you can use a few different techniques, such as disclosing solutions, drying the teeth, and using the explorer probe.

The use of the modified pen grasp is vital to the effectiveness of the hand instrument and protects the operator by reducing hand fatigue. The idea is to grip the instrument rather than pinch it. The handle of the instrument should be placed between the thumb and the index finger, with the middle finger on the shank of the instrument. The pinkie and the ring finger are then placed on or near the tooth being worked on to act as a fulcrum. A fulcrum is a place near the tooth that you are working on to support your hand. This creates stability and increases control of the instrument[2] (Fig. 5.9).

Use of the Hand Scaler

Hand scalers are for supragingival scaling only.[22] The sharp working tip can cause trauma to the gingiva. When using a scaler, you should always start at the gingival margin and move toward the crown. The sharp tip is for cleaning developmental grooves and fissures on the teeth. Hand scalers are also good for cleaning interdental spaces, as seen between the incisors.

Use of the Dental Curette

Curettes are used supra- and subgingivally, with their primary purpose being to remove subgingival calculus, plaque, and debris. Proper use of this instrument is imperative.

First, consider the way the instrument adapts to the tooth. The working end of the instrument is the last 1–2 mm of the tip or toe.[11] The working end is kept in contact with the tooth and is then adjusted to the changes of the contour of the tooth while

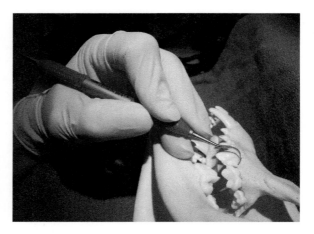

Figure 5.9   Modified pen grasp (Courtesy of John Koehm, DVM, FAVD).

cleaning.[2] This will assure that the surrounding tissues are not being damaged by the tip or toe of the instrument.

Subgingival scaling requires a different approach to angulation because curettes are inserted under the gum line. Gently insert the curette into the base of the pocket in a "closed" position. A closed position means that the face of the instrument is as close to 0 degrees as possible in relation to the tooth surface. Next, move the instrument to an open position so the angle of the face, in relation to the tooth, is at about 70 degrees. Again, while maintaining this angle and placing lateral pressure on the tooth during the stroke, you will achieve subgingival calculus removal.

When pulling the instrument, it is important to remember to rock your arm and wrist in the same motion and not to move just your fingers as this will cause great fatigue and result in long-term damage to your hands.

Disclosing Solution

Disclosing solution is a red dye that attaches to calculus and plaque. Although this is useful when you are beginning because it identifies areas that you missed, it is messy and will stain the patient, so should be used with great caution.

Dry the Teeth

Another way to see leftover debris is to dry the teeth with the air/water syringe on your machine. The calculus on the crown of the tooth will appear chalky white. Subgingival calculus will appear black. Your explorer can also help you detect calculus in areas that may not be easy to visualize.

Polishing

It is necessary to polish the teeth after scaling to remove any plaque left on the enamel surface. This also smooths etched enamel caused by scaling, without causing significant loss of enamel. Defects leave a rough surface on the enamel and create a hospitable environment for new plaque formation and retention.

Polishing is accomplished with a low-speed handpiece, a prophy angle with a prophy cup attached, and the correct paste. The low-speed handpiece can be either air driven or powered electrically with a motor pack. It should be run between 2000 and 4000 rpm to prevent too much heat from occurring while polishing. A good way to judge this is by running the handpiece at a comparable range and then trying to cause it to stop with your finger using gentle pressure. If it stalls, then you are fine. If you cannot stop it, your rpm's are too high. Use caution when doing this as you can easily burn your finger if there is too much friction.

There are two common types of prophy angles: standard circulating ones and oscillating ones. Circulating angles rotate a full 360 degrees, whereas oscillating angles move back and forth 90 degrees. Oscillating prophy angles are often preferred because they do not generate as much heat as circulating ones and because the patient's hair does not get caught in them.[6] Prophy angles are available in reusable metal and disposable plastic types. There are benefits to both types, and each practice will have a personal preference as to which type is used. Prophy cups are made of rubber and vary in their firmness. Soft-style prophy cups are preferred.[23] The softer cup requires less pressure for it to conform over the contours of the tooth surface and polish along the gingival margin.[3]

Prophy paste is needed to aid in polishing as well as to reduce friction on the tooth. Pastes vary in consistency, ranging from coarse to fine grit. Polishes that are coarse are typically used for stain removal, while fine-grit pastes are used for smoothing tooth surfaces. Some pastes are prepackaged individually and some are in bulk containers. Some pastes contain fluoride or glycerin; these should not be used if restorative dentistry is being performed.[6] Pastes can also cause artifacts on dental radiographs by showing up as little white flecks. Fine flour pumice mixed with water is often preferred and will not cause either of the above problems.[6]

When polishing teeth, be careful not to overheat the tooth. Hold the handpiece in a modified pen grasp and allow the prophy cup to pass over the tooth surface with little back and forth movement. Apply plenty of polish to each tooth because it reduces friction and smooths roughed surfaces. Move quickly over the tooth surface, spending only 3–5 seconds on each tooth. Use only enough pressure to cause the cup to flare open and be allowed to move just below the gum line.[10] Subgingival polishing is important to remove rough areas as well as plaque that can lead to attachment loss. When polishing subgingivally, remember to be very gentle so as not to injure the soft tissue.

After polishing is complete, irrigate the gingival sulcus and rinse the teeth and oral cavity. This is especially important when dealing with periodontal pockets as debris can be trapped in these areas, preventing healing.[23] This can be accomplished by using the air/water syringe on your dental unit as well as irrigation needles or curved tipped syringes with saline or a dilute chlorhexidine solution.

Air polishing is another technique available for polishing the teeth. It is done by spraying a combination of water and sodium bicarbonate on the tooth with a special handpiece that can attach either to a dental unit or a stand-alone machine. This is very technique sensitive and requires proper training. Incorrect nozzle angulation can cause damage to the gingival tissues, lips, cheeks, and tongue.[3] It is also important to protect yourself and the patient's eyes from the spray. Air polishing is beneficial for extrinsic stain removal as well as polishing areas that conventional polishing cannot reach, such as developmental grooves and interdental spaces (see web content: Video 5.2W Basics of the Dental Cleaning Part 2).[6]

Recovery

Once the dental procedure is complete, you can begin the patient recovery. Before ending the anesthesia, be sure to inspect the oral cavity for blood, debris, and excess water. Check for any loose debris between the lips, under the tongue, and in the back of the mouth. Rinse the oral cavity using your air/water syringe. Once you are sure that it is clean, remove the pharyngeal gauze pack and check again for debris in the area. You should also clean the head and face of any fluids and dry them. Take care to protect the patient's eyes and relubricate them as needed.

Because some patients may have a low body temperature after a dental procedure, some cleaning of the head and face may need to be done after their temperature has returned to normal. This is also a good time to check the intravenous catheter site for blood as it is easier to clean while the patient is still anesthetized.

Depending on the extent of the procedure, you may need to consider medications needed for recovery. If an extended painful procedure was performed, there might be a need for additional pain medications. (See Chapter 4 for further details.)

When ending general anesthesia, it is important to continue oxygen for several minutes as well as continue monitoring all vitals until the patient starts to show signs of recovery. These include the return of palpebral reflexes, eye position, jaw tone, changes in respiratory and heart rates, and swallowing reflexes. After several minutes, remove the patient from oxygen and challenge them on room air. Once the patient shows signs of recovery, you can start to remove some of the monitoring equipment, ideally, leaving at least one monitor on (i.e., Doppler or pulse oximeter). You should leave the endotracheal tube in place until the patient is swallowing. In brachycephalic breeds or animals with an elongated soft palate, you may need to leave the tube in place until the patient is almost completely recovered. Be sure to deflate the cuff before the patient begins to move to avoid any tracheal injury.

Once the endotracheal tube is removed, the patient can be moved to a recovery cage. The cage should be heated to help the patient maintain temperature during recovery. Continued patient monitoring for temperature and other vitals should be done every 30–60 minutes until the patient is fully recovered. Some patients will require continued pain management and fluid therapy for several hours or days. When appropriate, you may begin to offer the patient food and water and take them for a walk, allowing them to urinate.

Home Care

The goal of dental home care is to maintain a healthy oral environment and to prevent deterioration of previously existing periodontal disease.[24] This is attained by evaluating certain factors. First, learn how much the owner is committed or capable of doing at home. Second, evaluate the patient's level of disease and willingness to cooperate.[25]

The key to successful home care is owner education. The veterinary technician needs to help them understand the causes, effects, and means of prevention.

Plaque is a biofilm composed of bacteria, saliva, and food that forms on teeth shortly after a professional cleaning or brushing. The effects of plaque are halitosis, discomfort, and pain that can lead to chronic infection resulting in tooth loss. Other effects can be on the systemic level, causing renal and cardiac problems.[23] Prevention is now easier than ever before with the myriad of methods and products available. Helping the owner understand their responsibility in plaque control and prevention of periodontal disease will often help them perform good home care. This education should begin early so that the animal and the owner can learn together and continue over the life of the pet. The technician needs to help by monitoring progress and reinforcing the importance of consistent home care with the owner. It is also important to help them understand that even with good home care, professional exams and cleaning are necessary.

The technician, along with the entire staff, should be familiar with the products made available to owners. They should be able to discuss their use and benefits and demonstrate how to use them with confidence. When educating owners, it is good to have demonstration materials such as models, a demonstration dog or cat, handouts, and videos explaining the different methods of home care that are available. This will help them decide the best method for themselves and their pet.

Home care is broken into two different types: active and passive. Active home care is brushing, oral rinsing, or applying of barrier sealants. Passive home care is using diets, treats, chews, water additives, and dental sealants.[24,26]

Brushing is considered the gold standard of home care. There are times when this cannot be accomplished regularly due to the animal's behavior or the owner's inability or unwillingness to perform it. It is important to evaluate these factors early on so as not to cause the owner to get hurt or cause them to feel too pressured and disgruntled. This will also help the veterinarian decide the best course of treatment when performing a procedure.

If brushing is not an option, then oral rinses with a chlorhexidine or zinc base will help to a lesser degree. Another option is a barrier sealant application once a week. This may be more appealing to the client who will not commit to brushing but wants to do something. All of these active methods of home care keep the owner handling the mouth more aware of dental changes.

Passive forms of home care are often more attractive to owners. Dental diets are a common method of passive care. There are two diet formulations: chemical and mechanical. They are also categorized based on whether they work against plaque, calculus, or both. Chemical-based diets are often coated with sodium hexametaphosphate (SHMP). SHMP is a chelating agent that binds with calcium in the saliva, aiding in the prevention of calculus formation.[27] Diets that contain SHMP only work to prevent calculus and not plaque. However, by preventing calculus formation they are preventing larger surface areas for plaque to form on.

Mechanical diets are fiber-based diets that are designed to maximize the food's contact time on the tooth surface while the patient chews.[24] This shredding activity over the tooth surface actively disrupts plaque formation. Some diets combine both chemical and mechanical methods for maximum benefits.

Biscuit-type treats work in a similar manner to diets. They are often coated with SHMP and help control calculus but not plaque.[24] Chews such as Greenies® (The Nutro Company, Franklin, TN) are designed to mechanically control plaque and calculus by abrasion as the pet bites down on the chew. Rawhide chews are shown to help reduce plaque and calculus and to promote gingival health. It is important to differentiate between rawhide strips and pressed rawhide bones. These larger rawhides are much harder and place the pet at risk for dental fractures and possible foreign body. Some rawhide strips are also coated with SHMP to have additional calculus reduction. For current information on approved products, see VOHC.org (the website of the Veterinary Oral Health Council).[28]

Educating clients about proper chew toys is also important. Although chew toys are not proven to have a significant effect on plaque and calculus, they are widely used by owners. Chew toys such as Kong Balls® (Kong Company, Golden, CO) are designed to be safe for chewing without causing fractures. When choosing chew toys, it is important to consider the safety. Some criteria to use when selecting chews and toys are to see if it indents with your nail, softens with saliva, and is bendable. If the pet chews toys aggressively, toy play should be considered unsafe and should be monitored or a different toy chosen (see web content: Developing a Home Dental Health Care Plan).[28]

Brushing

Daily brushing is the best method for plaque control. Brushing every other day is also considered beneficial, but anything less than that is not effective in plaque, calculus, or gingivitis control.[4] Remember to start slowly and early in life.

Materials needed to be successful with brushing are a soft-bristled toothbrush, pet toothpaste, and a will to succeed. There are many different types of toothbrushes available. These include plastic finger brushes, smaller feline brushes, and dual-ended brushes. Finger brushes are a great tool for beginners; however, they are not ideal for long-term use. They are not as abrasive as a bristled brush and expose the owner to being bitten. Pet toothpastes have enzymatic properties that inhibit plaque formation, but more importantly, they are flavored, so the pet will accept them. Because pets swallow toothpaste, human toothpaste cannot be used due to gastrointestinal upset caused by the detergents. It is important to emphasize that the mechanical action of brushing helps control plaque.[29]

Be patient; it can take weeks to months to be able to brush effectively. Start slowly and be gentle. It is helpful to place the pet up on a couch, chair, or counter for smaller animals. This puts them at your level and gives you more control of the situation. Create a daily pattern for you and the pet. Start giving the toothpaste at the same time and place and by the same person every day. This causes the pet to anticipate the toothpaste as a treat. Before long, they will be looking forward to their treat. While giving them the toothpaste, touch the face and muzzle. Begin lifting the lips and rubbing the gums and teeth. This will begin to desensitize them. It is not necessary to force the mouth open. You can then start to place the toothpaste on the brush and allow them to lick it while continuing to manipulate to face as described. Introduce the brush, starting in the front of the mouth at the incisors and canines. With gradual acceptance, increase the number of teeth brushed, advancing further back in the mouth to the premolars then the molars.[29] It is important to remember that the maxillary molars angle in toward the midline and you will need to change your brushing angle to accommodate this. On the mandible, the overlap of the upper fourth premolar and the lower first molar causes a need for you to open the mouth slightly when brushing. Sometimes placing a toy in the mouth helps to accomplish this. Move the brush in a circular or side-to-side motion at a 45-degree angle to the tooth surface. The bristles at the tooth and gum margin should be angled to engage the gingival sulcus with the emphasis on the stroke away from the gum line.[30] A complete brushing will last about 2 minutes or about 30 seconds per quadrant[29] (Fig. 5.10). A useful video demonstration can be seen at https://www.youtube.com/watch?v=B_E5Uuf-JCY (see web content: Brushing the Teeth).

See Appendix 1 for home oral health care interview form.

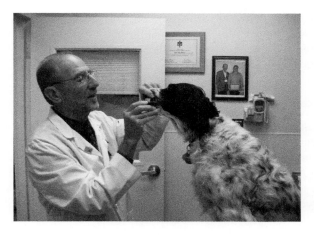

Figure 5.10   Using a demonstration dog to help educate owners on how to brush teeth (Courtesy of John Koehm, DVM, FAVD).

Equipment and Instrument Care

Power scalers need to have the stacks, rods, and tips checked regularly. Bent or fractured stacks cannot tune and spray water correctly. This results in increased heat and decreased effectiveness of the instrument. Piezoelectric and sonic tips have guides that help you determine when it is too worn to be effective.

Compressors need to have the oil checked and changed (follow manufacturer recommendations). They also have air and water filters that need to be cleaned or changed. The fan should also be cleaned regularly. If there is an air tank, it should be drained of condensation.

Instrument Sharpening

Sharpening scalers and curettes is a necessity. To check for instrument sharpness, use an acrylic rod and engage the cutting edge of the instrument on the rod. If it is sharp, it will shave a thin slice off the stick.[5] If it is dull, it will not engage the stick well and will skip over the surface. You can also visually inspect the instrument by holding it in the light. If the edges reflect the light, they are dull. Make sure that the instruments are cleaned before sharpening to avoid contaminating the stones, and then cleaned and sterilized after sharpening to remove any sharpening remnants. This is to ensure that you do not contaminate your stones and to protect the patient from sharpening remnants.

Sharpening equipment

To begin sharpening, you need a sharpening stone. There are several types, but there are a few standard ones that are needed. First is a fine Arkansas stone for regular sharpening. Next is an India stone which is coarser and used on dull instruments or to recontour instruments. The last one is a conical stone and is used to sharpen the face of the instrument. All three types require oil during sharpening. Ceramic stones are also available that do not require oil for sharpening. The Rx Honing machine

(The Rx Honing Machine Corp., Mishawaka, IN; www.rxhoning.com) is also available. It has guides that provide the correct angles for sharpening curettes and scalers while a mounted stone rotates on a mandrel.[7] It is technique sensitive and must be used with caution.

Sharpening technique

One common sharpening technique is the stationary instrument/moving stone. Place oil on the stone and disperse it evenly. Next, hold the instrument on a counter edge with the instrument face parallel to the floor and the tip facing you. Then hold the stone in the opposite hand between your thumb and forefinger on the top and the bottom of the stone. Place the stone parallel to the instrument the angle it away about 15 degrees. This will put the stone at either an 11 o'clock or 1 o'clock position. While maintaining the correct angle, move the stone up and down two to three short strokes, ending on a downward stroke. If the instrument is a universal instrument, then repeat on the other side. For a curette, the stone is rotated around the front of the instrument to keep the blunt toe shape. As a final step, take the conical stone and roll it along the face of the instrument to remove any spurs that might have formed on the edges (see web content: Figs. 5.11W and 5.12W).[5]

References

1. Holmstrom, S, Bellows, J, Colmery, B, Conway, L, Knutson, K, Vitoux, J. 2005. AAHA dental care guidelines for dogs and cats. *Journal of the American Animal Hospital Association* 41:277–283.
2. Wilkins, EM. 2009. *Clinical Practice of the Dental Hygienist*, 10th edn. Philadelphia, PA: Lippincott Williams & Wilkins.
3. Nield-Gehrig, J. 2008. *Fundamentals of Periodontal Instrumentation and Advanced Root Instrumentation*, 6th edn. Philadelphia, PA: Lippincott Williams & Wilkins.
4. Mitchell, PQ. 2002. Periodontics. In *The Practical Veterinarian: Small Animal Dentistry*. Boston, MA: Butterworth-Heinemann, pp. 59–103.
5. Wiggs, RB, Lobprise, HB. 1997. Dental equipment. In *Veterinary Dentistry: Principles and Practice*. Philadelphia, PA: Lippincott-Raven, pp. 1–28.
6. Holmstrom, S. 2000. The complete prophy. In *Veterinary Dentistry for the Technician and Office Staff*. Philadelphia, PA: WB Saunders, pp. 159–181.
7. Holmstrom, SE, Frost Fitch, P, Eisner, ER. 2004. Dental equipment and care. In *Veterinary Dental Techniques for the Small Animal Practitioner*, 3rd edn. Philadelphia, PA: WB Saunders, pp. 30–129.
8. American Veterinary Dental College. Abbreviations for use in AVDC case logs, https://avdc.org/wp-content/uploads/2019/08/abbreviations.pdf (accessed March, 2020).
9. Holmstrom, S. 2000. Introduction. In *Veterinary Dentistry for the Technician and Office Staff*. Philadelphia, PA: WB Saunders, pp. 1–22.
10. Kessel, LM. 2000. Performing the dental prophy. In *Veterinary Dentistry for the Small Animal Technician*. Ames, IA: Iowa State University Press, pp. 81–99.
11. Newman, MG, Takel, HH, Carranza, FA. 2002. *Carranza's Clinical Pathology*, 9th edn. Philadelphia, PA: Lippincott Williams & Wilkins.

CHAPTER 5

12. Gorrel, C. 2004. Oral examination and recording. In *Veterinary Dentistry for the General Practitioner*. Philadelphia, PA: Elsevier, pp. 47–55.
13. Wiggs, RB, Lobprise, HB. 1997. Oral anatomy and physiology. In *Veterinary Dentistry: Principles and Practice*. Philadelphia, PA: Lippincott-Raven, pp. 55–86.
14. Lobprise, HB. 2007. Oral exam and charting. In *Blackwell's Five-Minute Consult Clinical Companion Small Animal Dentistry*. Ames, IA: Blackwell Publishing, pp. 3–13.
15. Hale, F. 2008. Focus on: gingival hyperplasia. http://toothvet.ca/PDFfiles/gingival_hyperplasia.pdf (accessed March, 2020).
16. American Veterinary Dental College. Tooth mobility. https://avdc.org/avdc-nomenclature/ (accessed March, 2020).
17. American Veterinary Dental College. Furcation involvement/exposure. https://avdc.org/avdc-nomenclature/ (accessed March, 2020).
18. Holmstrom, S. 2000. The oral exam and disease recognition. In *Veterinary Dentistry for the Technician and Office Staff*. Philadelphia, PA: WB Saunders, pp. 23–64.
19. Lobprise, HB. 2007. Tooth resorption: feline. In *Blackwell's Five-Minute Consult Clinical Companion Small Animal Dentistry*. Ames, IA: Blackwell Publishing, pp. 309–313.
20. Gorrel, C. 2004. Common oral conditions. In *Veterinary Dentistry for the General Practitioner*. Philadelphia, PA: Elsevier, pp. 69–85.
21. Hale, F. 2004. Dental caries. www.toothvet.ca/PDFfiles/DentalCaries.pdf ().
22. Holmstrom, S. 2000. Dental instruments and equipment. In *Veterinary Dentistry for the Technician and Office Staff*. Philadelphia, PA: WB Saunders, pp. 65–98.
23. Gorrel, C. 2004. Periodontal disease. In *Veterinary Dentistry for the General Practitioner*. Philadelphia, PA: Elsevier, pp. 87–110.
24. Roudebush, P, Logan, E, Hale, FA. 2005. Evidence-based veterinary dentistry: a systemic review of homecare for prevention of periodontal disease in dogs and cats. *Journal of Veterinary Dentistry* 22:6–15.
25. Hale, F. 2003. The owner-animal-environment triad in the treatment of canine periodontal disease. *Journal of Veterinary Dentistry* 20:118–122.
26. Holmstrom, S. 2000. Home care instructions. In *Veterinary Dentistry for the Technician and Office Staff*. Philadelphia, PA: WB Saunders, pp. 65–98.
27. Bellows, J. 2010. Clinical effectiveness of sodium hexametaphosphate in the important role of canine calculus reduction. https://s3.amazonaws.com/assets.prod.vetlearn.com/4c/63ee70296811e0a58a0050568d634f/file/VT10044%20Hartz%20White%20Paper%207-28-1.pdf (accessed March, 2020).
28. Veterinary Oral Health Council. Products currently awarded the VOHC seal. www.vohc.org/accepted_products.htm (accessed August 29, 2010).
29. Berg, M. 2005. Educating clients about preventative dentistry. *Veterinary Technician* 26:103–111.
30. Wiggs, RB, Lobprise, HB. 1997. Periodontology. In *Veterinary Dentistry: Principles and Practice*. Philadelphia, PA: Lippincott-Raven, pp. 186–231.

Dentaical Radiology

6

Laurel Bird, CVT, VTS (Dentistry)

Learning Objectives

- Describe the position of the sensor, phosphor plates, or film in the feline mouth to take radiographs of the maxillary incisors, mandibular incisors/mandibular canine teeth, maxillary canine teeth, maxillary premolars/molars, and mandibular premolars/molars
- Describe the position of the sensor, phosphor plates, or film in the canine mouth to take radiographs of the maxillary incisors, mandibular incisors/mandibular canine teeth, maxillary canine teeth, maxillary premolars/molars, and mandibular premolars/molars
- Determine proper orientation of a dental image: maxilla versus mandible, left versus right
- Identify a diagnostic image
- Identify normal radiographic structures

Small Animal Dental Procedures for Veterinary Technicians and Nurses, Second Edition.
Edited by Jeanne R. Perrone.
© 2021 John Wiley & Sons, Inc. Published 2021 by John Wiley & Sons, Inc.

CHAPTER 6

Radiography in Veterinary Dentistry

Radiography in veterinary dentistry is invaluable in identifying pathology that cannot be observed with the naked eye within the oral cavity. Without its use, much pathology may go undetected by the veterinary team. Teeth that appear normal on the surface may be suffering from any number of pathological events that can only be detected using dental radiographs. Some of the pathology that it is used to identify is endodontic disease, periodontal bone loss, and the extent of damage from tooth resorption, in addition to unerupted teeth and jaw fractures, to name just a few.[1,2] The value of dental radiography should never be underestimated and must be part of every dental procedure. In addition, the American Animal Hospital Association (AAHA) Dental Care Guidelines for Dogs and Cats state that preoperative and postoperative dental radiographs are mandated for all extractions.[3]

Some issues veterinarians have with taking dental radiographs are added anesthesia time and radiation exposure due to radiograph retakes because images were not of diagnostic quality on the first take (elongation, foreshortening, poor alignment with area in question, over/underprocessing, improper machine settings). Care should be taken when producing images to minimize these errors that require retakes, for the safety of the pet and personnel. Ideally, a diagnostic image should be accomplished on the first take. Although the process of obtaining dental radiographs adds anesthesia time, the wealth of information obtained far outweighs the risk for many patients.

Patients with increased anesthetic risk can be referred to a veterinary dental specialist where procedures can be accomplished in a minimal time and advanced anesthetic care may be provided by some clinics. Many times, recommendations can be made prior to anesthesia for evaluations by cardiologists, internal medicine, or other specialists to provide more information about the patient's health. In addition, some veterinary clinics and hospitals have access to technicians with specialties in anesthesia and veterinary anesthesiologists. This may allow some patients previously thought to be unable to undergo anesthesia, to receive treatment and alleviate the pain and infection of dental disease safely.

The veterinary technician is a great person to be delegated the task of taking dental radiographs for the veterinarian. The techniques necessary are well within the scope of a technician's skillset and most technicians can learn how to produce diagnostic images with practice. In this chapter you will learn how to use the dental X-ray unit, how to use a digital sensor, phosphor plates, or film, and how to identify a diagnostic image.

The Dental X-Ray Unit

Veterinary technicians are familiar with how to operate a standard X-ray machine and the dental X-ray unit is not much different, mechanically speaking. The standard medical X-ray unit has adjustable milliamp (mA), peak kilovoltage (kVp), and time settings.[4] However, the fixed or limited range-of-motion tube head reduces its usefulness in dentistry. Although dental radiographs can be taken with a standard medical X-ray unit, the difficulties in moving the patient, positioning them for intraoral films, and adjusting the machine make it unlikely that a practice could rely on this as a method for taking dental images.

Dental X-ray units offer many benefits to the practice of veterinary dentistry and are useful for radiographs of other small structures or patients. The dental X-ray unit is relatively inexpensive, compact, flexible, and easy to use. New or used units can be obtained through a variety of suppliers. The unit can be wall-mounted next to the station(s) where it will be used, then folded up to be relatively flat against a wall when not in use. Otherwise, it can be mounted on a wheeled cart which allows the unit to be moved to different locations for use, then wheeled to an out of the way corner for storage. There are even portable hand-held X-ray units that are used in veterinary dentistry.

There are three main parts to the standard dental X-ray unit: the X-ray tube head, the adjustable arm, and the control panel (Fig. 6.1). Portable units do not have an adjustable arm and have the control panel and tube head combined in one hand-held device.

The X-Ray Tube Head

The X-ray tube head contains the anode/cathode that generates the X-rays. It includes a scale located where the head attaches to the arm that can be used to determine various angles (Fig. 6.2). The focal film distance is measured using the

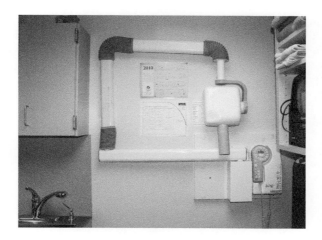

Figure 6.1 Wall-mounted X-ray unit.

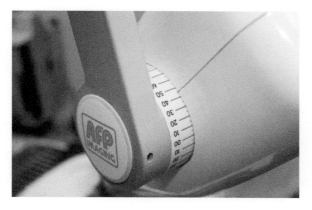

Figure 6.2 Scale used to determine X-ray tube head position for radiographs. It is set at 45 degrees.

lead-lined tube or position indicating device (PID) and provides collimation that will result in less scattered radiation. The PID comes in a variety of lengths and moving the PID closer or further from the patient will also change the focal film distance. The best practice is to keep the end of the PID as close to the patient and plate/sensor as possible without touching the patient. This allows most of the radiation to contact the plate/sensor with minimal magnification or scatter.

The Adjustable Arm

The adjustable arm is just that – an arm that can be adjusted in a wide array of angles and levels to position the X-ray tube head, so radiation is directed at the plate/sensor. It contains adjustable screws to allow you to tighten or loosen the tension on the arm to prevent drift once positioned. Over time, they may need adjustment. If you position your tube head and it drifts or moves once you let go, it is time to adjust the tension screws. Consult the manufacturer for instruction on how to perform this for each different model.

The Control Panel

The control panel contains the settings for the unit. In many units the peak kilovoltage is fixed, as is the milliamperage, eliminating the need for some adjustments to the settings. Time is usually the main setting that needs to be adjusted and many units make even that measurement simple by providing small, medium and large canine settings or a feline setting and then a pictogram of the animal oral cavity allowing you to select the tooth being radiographed (Fig. 6.3). This is essentially two buttons

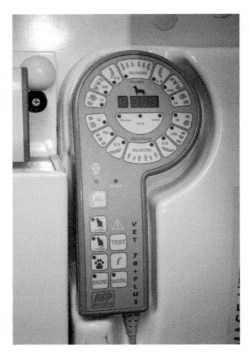

Figure 6.3   The control panel of a typical veterinary dental X-ray unit.

to push to set the unit for taking a radiograph. Should you have a unit with adjustable peak kilovoltage and/or milliamperage then a technique chart can be created as you would for any other X-ray machine. Most units can operate on 110 V, 60 Hz AC electricity, although a separate electrical circuit is usually required.

Just a few comments about safety when using dental X-ray units: Personnel throughout the clinic should be aware of and follow all standard radiation safety protocols. Everyone should always be 6 feet (2 m) or more from the tube head, at an angle of 90–135 degrees to the beam, or should wear lead-lined equipment to minimize radiation exposure. Wearing a dosimeter badge will also help check for inadvertent exposure. The sensor, plate, or film should never be held by hand in the animal's mouth by anyone (lead gloves or not). Finally, the unit should be checked regularly for radiation leakage by a radiation expert; many states have regulations to help you set up a schedule of inspection.[5]

Dental Radiographic Image Media and Capture

Various media for capturing dental radiographic images are available. Film was the original medium, but digital sensors and phosphor plates have become commonplace. Although these three media differ slightly in appearance and use, all produce an image, albeit with varying degree of clarity; digital images are typically clearer than film. All media use a standard dental X-ray generator although the settings will vary.

Digital imagery has an initial higher cost for the sensor or phosphor plates and software. Advantages, however, include the lower radiation needed to produce an image, immediately available images with quick retake ability (should the image not be appropriate for a diagnosis), and images that can be manipulated using a computer (for better viewing and enhancement of structures).[5] Most digital software for sensors and phosphor plates will allow photos to be imported so pictures of oral masses and other pathology can be easily stored with the radiographic images. This is a great way to store those before-the-procedure and after-the-procedure photos for easy recall.

The larger phosphor plates/size 4 film are useful for imaging larger areas of the oral cavity involved in dentigerous cysts, oral tumors, and fractures. Although it is not necessary to have the entire tooth on a single image, some may prefer to examine them this way and thus choose to use larger phosphor plates or size 4 film. These are also useful for nondental radiographs of feline paws, pocket pets and other exotics and even neonatal patients for a variety of purposes.

Care should be taken to produce a radiographically diagnostic image on the first attempt in order to minimize patient and staff exposure to radiation as well as minimize patient time under anesthesia.

Ensure that the structure of interest is on the image either in its entirety or as much of it as possible. Two or more images may be necessary for larger teeth and multirooted teeth as well as nontooth structures.

The structure should contain minimal or no foreshortening or elongation and should be representative of the structure being radiographed. The tooth should look like the tooth in the mouth and be proportionately similar. Foreshortening and elongation can hide or accentuate pathology and must be avoided, allowing the best opportunity to diagnose problems.

Every tooth root being evaluated should have 2–3 mm of normal bone visible surrounding them on an image. If other structures are being radiographed, they require the same 2–3 mm of normal tissue around the structure of interest. Cutting off this surrounding bone too close at the edge of the image may cause pathology to be missed or underdiagnosed.

Contrast and brightness should be correct on the image. If the image is too dark (overexposed) or too light (underexposed), adjustments to the settings should be made and a retake performed. An overexposed image will prevent viewing of thinner structures such as alveolar bone, smaller tooth crowns, etc. as they will be burned through or appear black in areas that have normal structure. Although some lightening of the image may be performed with the program software in the case of digital images, if the original image is overexposed it is likely that some structures will be hidden. An underexposed image will be too light and be difficult to evaluate. Structures will have a lack of contrast (black/white/grays) and there is often a foggy appearance to the overall image.

Reading the Dental Radiographic Image[5]

Intraoral images should be viewed in labial presentation. Imagine that the animal was standing in front of you and you are looking at the teeth. This is labial presentation – viewing the teeth from the labial (lip) aspect of the animal. Maxillary teeth should be viewed with crowns pointing downward and mandibular teeth viewed with crowns pointed upward.

To determine correct or labial presentation on a digital image, first identify maxillary versus mandibular structures, then determine if the image is of the left or right arcade. Most digital software will orient the image correctly if the sensor or phosphor plate is placed in the mouth according to the manufacturer's recommendations and the correct teeth were selected in the software prior to taking the image. However, it is useful to know how to correctly orient an image and recognize maxilla or mandible should the image be rotated the wrong way.

First, determine whether the image is of maxilla or mandible. Structures that can help determine a maxillary tooth include visibility of the palatine fissures on incisor images or nasal passages and sinuses on other views, a visible radiodense white line along the apices of the tooth roots (this is the nasal surface of the alveolar process of the maxilla),[5] and lack of mandibular structures (Fig. 6.4). Mandibular teeth are determined by the visibility of the mandibular symphysis, mandibular canal, or ventral cortex of the mandible (Fig. 6.5). You may need to rotate the image if the crowns of the teeth are not pointing in the correct direction as noted earlier (Fig. 6.6).

Next, determine left or right arcade of the animal. If oriented correctly as discussed in the previous two paragraphs, incisor views will have the animal's right teeth on your left side and vice versa. The lateral views of the teeth on the right arcades will have the canine tooth to your right and the molars will be to your left. The lateral view of the teeth on the left arcades will have the canine tooth on the left and molars on the right.

Correctly orienting film images will take an extra step. Your first task will be to view the correct side of the film. This is done by making sure the raised side of the dot in the corner of each film is facing you (Fig. 6.7). After that, you follow the instructions given earlier for identifying maxilla/mandible and then right/left.

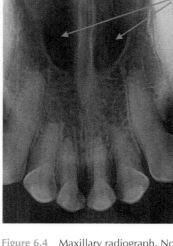 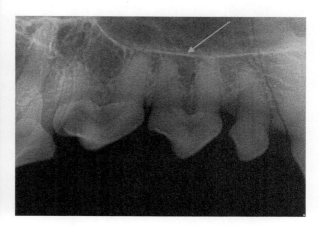

Figure 6.4   Maxillary radiograph. Note the palatine fissures (red arrows) on the left image and the white line of the nasal surface of the alveolar process of the maxilla along the roots of the premolars (blue arrow) on the right image.

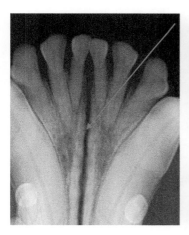 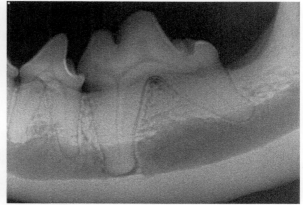

Figure 6.5   Mandibular radiograph. Note the mandibular symphysis (red arrow) on the left image. The right image has the mandibular canal and ventral cortex of the mandible visible and a lack of maxillary structures.

It is important that you are able to identify the radiographic appearance of each tooth in the mouth. Practice identifying the look of first, second, and third incisors. Whether maxillary or mandibular, they each have a specific silhouette. The same applies to first, second, third, and fourth premolars and each of the molars. Canine teeth are generally easy to identify on radiographs, but the other teeth may require you to practice identifying each tooth and tooth type. Many vets and techs find it helpful to have a skull present to match up what they are seeing in the radiograph with the physical structures on the skull (Fig. 6.8).

It is critical that you are able to correctly identify which teeth are being examined in order to avoid mistakes in treating teeth.

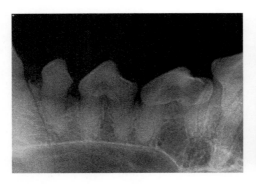 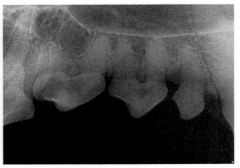

Figure 6.6 The image on the left is a radiograph of a maxillary arcade with the crowns pointing in the wrong direction. The image on the right is of the same radiograph correctly oriented. Note the white line along the tooth roots that alerts us to the fact that these are maxillary teeth and thus the image needed to be rotated.

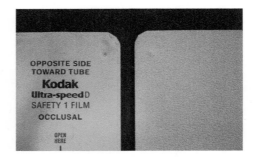

Figure 6.7 Film dot, back and front of film packet. The film itself will have this same raised area.

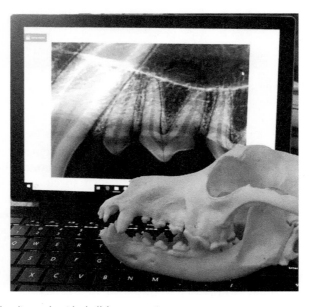

Figure 6.8 Dental radiograph with skull for comparison.

The Digital Sensor

Sensors come in limited sizes, with the most common being equivalent to film size 2 (this is the largest size of sensor currently available), and generally have a cable attaching them to a computer (Fig. 6.9). A new thin plastic, hygienic sheath should be used on the sensor and changed after each patient to prevent cross-contamination and to keep the sensor dry. Larger teeth will need two or more views/images to see the whole tooth.

Although most sensors are similar, their software will vary, and it is important that you know how to use as many features of the software as possible. This allows you to get the most out of your system. Some allow you to take a radiograph and view/adjust the image all from one screen. Others require you to exit the acquisition mode and go to a different part of the software to manipulate the image. Most software allows you to take images in a template, which is helpful in viewing radiographs and making sure you have imaged all portions of every tooth (Fig. 6.10). Be sure to identify each set of radiographs at the start, with owner/patient name and date. Try to use unique identifiers such as birthdate of pet and/or the practice management software client/patient ID numbers/letters. Over time you will encounter many pets and owners with similar names and it is imperative that you are able to select the correct patient each time.

Most software will allow you to store images sets from each date under the same patient and yet view different years at the same time. Another feature you may find in your software is searchable databases for specific tooth numbers or specific dates. This is handy as over the years you will have patients that have large numbers of radiographs from different dental procedures.

The ability to download and email radiographs is also very helpful in sharing images with other veterinarians or specialists. Most software has this ability.

When capturing the image, the smooth, flat side of the sensor is placed in the mouth facing the teeth to be radiographed. The teeth are selected in the software and, once exposed to radiation, the image is sent to a computer for immediate viewing.

Note that animals being radiographed with sensors should be fully anesthetized, not just sedated, so they do not accidentally bite down on the sensor. Bites to the sensor are the most common causes of damage that results in sensor replacement, followed by being dropped, stepped on, or crushed. Bites on the sensor can cause anything from one or two pixels being damaged to the entire sensor failing. Damaged sensors result in delayed procedures as you wait for a replacement unless you have

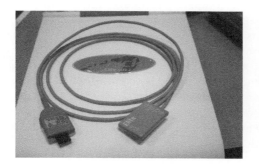

Figure 6.9   Digital sensor.

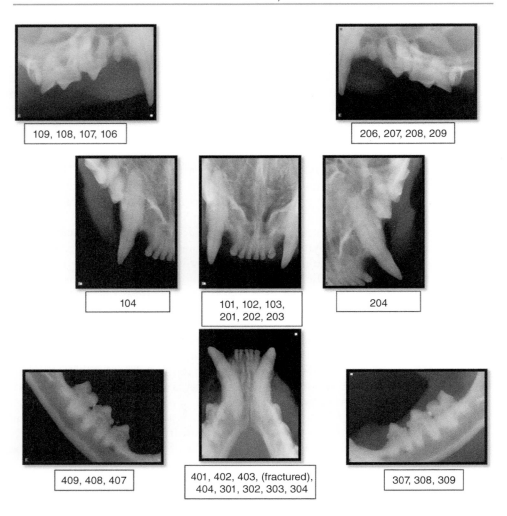

Figure 6.10 Template showing all dentition in a cat.

another method for capturing radiographic dental images. Care should also be taken to protect the sensor's cable from crimping or crushing as well to prevent similar issues. Sensors can be costly to replace as well as causing delayed procedures.

Once loaded into the computer, the image contrast, brightness, and sharpness can be changed. The image can also be enlarged to assist in reading it. Most systems have other adjustments as well to enhance various structures on the image and these will vary by manufacturer (Fig. 6.11).

Rotating an image is a common option. Rotating an image will spin it like the hands on a clock and can be useful if the tooth's orientation is not correct, as can happen when the wrong tooth is selected in the software. Do not flip an image side to side or top to bottom. Because there is no dot or other mark on most system images to help orient directions, flipping an image can cause interpretation errors and the wrong tooth may be treated.

Advantages of sensors versus film include ease of use (short learning curve for most people as the sensor is left in place until an image is evaluated for diagnostic

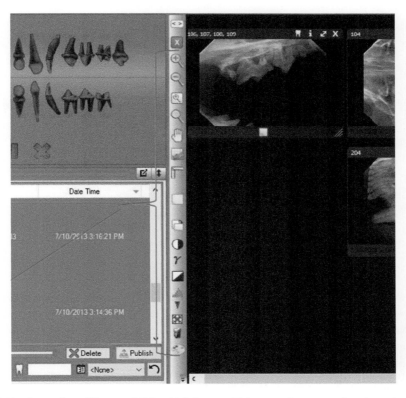

Figure 6.11   Screenshot of Progeny (Midmark) Software with image enhancement bar down the center (red bracket).

quality), a digital image that allows easy retrieval, electronic transfer of images, computer enhancement, and no chemicals.

Disadvantages over film include higher upfront cost, the need for a computer to view images on, and digital storage for images. Sensors will need to be replaced eventually but most last for years if well cared for and some veterinarians will replace a sensor primarily to get updated technology. Most people agree the advantages of sensors over film far outweigh the disadvantages.

Phosphor Plate Radiographs

Phosphor plates combine the versatility of film sizes with the convenience of digital images. The phosphor plate is thin, like film, placed in a protective plastic sleeve, and then used the same as dental film (Fig. 6.12).

Phosphor plates are placed in the mouth with the back side of the plate (the side without writing on it) toward the teeth to be radiographed. Always check manufacturer's recommendations. Once the tooth is selected in the software, the exposure is taken and the plate is removed from the mouth. It is then loaded into a special machine that "develops" or processes the image, digitalizing it and transferring it to a computer. Once on the computer, the image can be viewed and manipulated in the same way as other digital images. The processor also erases the plate, so it is ready to be placed in a new sleeve and used again.

CHAPTER 6

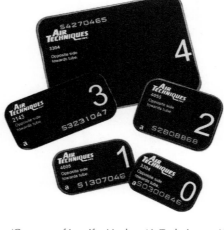

Figure 6.12   Phosphor plates (Courtesy of Jennifer Healey, Air Techniques, Allpro Imaging).

As with sensors, phosphor plate software will vary between manufacturers. Again, they will allow the basic adjustments of rotation in case the image orientation is incorrect, as well as contrast, brightness, and sharpness. Most allow the use of templates, email capabilities, and importing of photos. Be sure to explore your software to get the most out of your system.

Note that animals being radiographed with phosphor plates should be fully anesthetized, not just sedated, so they do not accidentally bite down on the phosphor plate. Bites to the plate are a common cause of damage that results in scratches or bends in the plate. Scratches and bends or bend marks in a plate will cause defects in the digital image that can make interpretation difficult. Damaged plates result in delayed procedures as you wait for a replacement, though most clinics using phosphor plates have 2–3 of each size used. It may mean a prolonged procedure time as images need to be processed before the plate(s) are available for the next image. Plates can be costly to replace as well as causing delays in procedures.

Although each plate will eventually need to be replaced, most systems allow for hundreds of images per plate. The cost of replacing phosphor plates is more than a box of film, but is significantly less than replacing a sensor.

Phosphor plates will require higher radiation settings than a sensor. Although the time setting is generally higher than used with sensors, it is still less than needed for film and again, time is typically the only adjustment most people use.

Advantages of phosphor plates include the ease of use, versatility from varied plate sizes, reusable plates in a variety of sizes, and a digital image that allows easy retrieval, electronic transfer of the image, computer enhancement, and no chemicals.

Disadvantages of phosphor plates over film include the higher upfront cost of a processing unit and plates and the need for a computer for viewing images and digital storage of images. The learning curve is similar to film. Most agree that, like sensors, the advantages far outweigh to disadvantages.

The advantages and disadvantages of sensors versus phosphor plates are mostly personal preference. Both take clear images and allow all the perks of digital images and software. The learning curve may be slightly greater for some individuals with a phosphor plate as it is removed from the mouth for processing. If positioning is an issue, you may have difficulty exactly replicating the original placement in the mouth, making adjustments more of a challenge. However, the versatility of different plate sizes may outweigh this disadvantage for some people.

Dental Film and Processing

Dental X-ray films are inexpensive, nonscreened, direct exposure films that provide good detail and come in several different speeds (this refers to the amount of radiation required to produce an image). Fast film equals less radiation, though it gives a grainier image, with A film being the slowest and F being the fastest. Film speeds A–C are not used due to the higher radiation needed to produce an image. D-speed film is the most commonly used film in veterinary dentistry. E speed film is available. All film uses more radiation than either sensors or phosphor plates.

Dental film comes in a variety of sizes, though most clinics find that size 0, 2, and 4 films work best for most canine and feline radiographs. Some manufacturers or suppliers may use other terminology when referring to dental film. For instance, size 0 film may also be noted as DF-54 or pediatric, size 2 film may be DF-58 or periapical film, and size 4 may be DF-50 or occlusal film if using D-speed film. The film should be kept in a dark, cool, dry location protected from radiation exposure until needed. Each film is used just once (Fig. 6.13).

There are four parts to the dental X-ray film packet. The outside is a paper or plastic coating to protect the film from moisture and has a white front side with a raised dot in one corner to assist in orienting the film once it is developed and a colored back side. The colored side will let you know if the packet contains one (green back, Kodak, Carestream, Rochester, NY) or two films (gray back, Kodak). Different manufacturers may use different color schemes so be sure to check with your manufacturer if there is any question.

The white side is always placed toward the teeth being radiographed. Once exposed, the packet is removed from the mouth and opened only in a darkroom or inside a chairside developing box. The packet is opened from the colored side; there is a lead foil sheet to prevent radiation scatter that could affect the film image. Black paper surrounds and protects the film, and the film itself is in the center (Fig. 6.14). Some manufacturers combine the lead and inner paper layers, especially for the large size 4 films. Note: The thin lead sheets should not be thrown in the garbage in most communities but should be sent to a lead recycler.

Dental film is processed in either a manual chairside developer or an automatic processor. Care must be taken when developing and handling films as they are easily

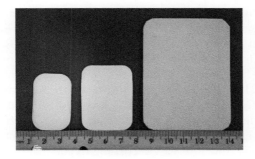

Figure 6.13   Assorted film sizes. Shown here are, from left to right, size 0, 2, and 4.

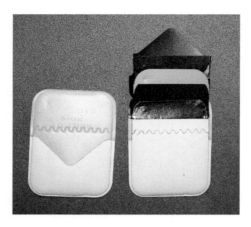

Figure 6.14   Dental film packet with protective outer barrier, black paper, film (green), and lead sheet.

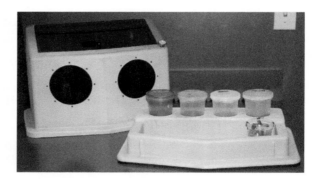

Figure 6.15   Chairside developing unit with cups for chemicals (from left to right): developer, rinse water, fixer, and final rinse water.

scratched, especially when wet. Although some people have tried to use standard film processors for their dental films, it is not recommended as the smaller dental films may become "lost" or stuck to the rollers. There are automatic processors available specifically for dental film and are used similarly to standard processors. These can be purchased through most equipment suppliers and manufacturer's instructions followed for the unit.

If you are using a manual chairside developer, it is still relatively quick and easy to produce a quality diagnostic image. Chairside developers are compact, light-tight boxes that allow you to develop film close to where you take the radiographs. Films can generally be ready to read in as little as 1–2 minutes, although they will not be dry. The chairside developer box has two hand holes on the front side with fitted cuffs to keep light out. The top side of the box has a translucent orange or red light-filtering lid. This allows you to see what you are doing inside the box without risking light exposure to the film. The orange filter is used for D-film and the red filter is used for E- and F- speed film. Inside the box are four cups; from left to right they contain developer, water for a rinse, fixer, and water for the final rinse (Fig. 6.15). The film is passed from one cup to the other from left to right at specific time intervals according to chemical and film manufacturer directions.

To develop films manually, gently mix each cup of developer and fixer and change the rinse water for fresh, cool water at the beginning of the developing session. Ensure that the filter cover is firmly seated, so no light leaks in. Insert hands and film through the cuffed openings, working with one film at a time. Open the film packet and place a film clip in the corner; many people place the clip in the corner with the indent. Gently agitate or swish film in the developer for the given time frame. Move the film to the first rinse cup and gently agitate for 1 minute to rinse excess developer from the film. The film can then be placed in the fixer cup and agitated occasionally. The film should remain in the fixer for at least 10 minutes for a long-lasting image, although you can briefly remove the film from the fixer and view the image after 1–2 minutes. Just be sure to immediately return the film to the fixer for the full time. The film must then be thoroughly rinsed for 10–20 minutes in the final rinse cup or, preferably, under running water to remove all chemical traces. You can gently rub the X-ray to help remove chemical traces; they will feel nongreasy when completely rinsed. Be careful not to scratch the films when rubbing them. Allow films to dry completely without touching other films or objects as they will stick together. Timing is important to receive a quality, lasting image, so close attention is needed.

Chemical developer and fixer can be purchased through most veterinary distributors and generally come premixed. Follow your local regulations when disposing of the chemical.

Note: Check your chairside developer box in the location you plan to use it. Although the filter tops are designed to keep light out, the bright overhead lights in clinics may require you to move the unit to a slightly darker location. Testing can be accomplished by placing a dental film in the box and opening and exposing a quarter of the film at 30-second intervals; then develop as usual. Any fogging of the film will alert you to light penetration.

Advantages of film over digital images are versatility in the size of films, though this is minimal as phosphor plates also offer a similar variety of sizes.

Disadvantages include increased radiation needs, an image that is not digital, and no access to computer enhancements (cannot adjust contrast, brightness, or sharpness unless you retake the film, nor can you enlarge the image for better viewing). It is hard to share films as they must be mailed or transported by the client to other vets or specialists, increasing the risk of lost or misplaced portions of a medical record. In addition, the time to take, develop, view, and retake films, if needed, is significantly longer even over phosphor plates. The chemicals can be messy to work with and disposal is a concern in some communities. Storage is an issue as well, since film occupies physical space and must be kept cool and dry both before and after use.

Most will agree that the disadvantages of using film are significant and a digital option should be chosen.

Positioning for Taking Dental Radiographs

Intraoral radiographs are the most common form of dental radiographs used in veterinary dentistry and taking quality intraoral images is a skill all veterinary technicians should master. Animals being radiographed should be fully anesthetized, not just sedated, so they do not inadvertently bite down on the sensor, plate, or film.

Depending on which media you choose, the cost of replacement can be expensive, and this simple step can extend the life of sensors or plates.

Positioning is a skill that will require practice to achieve competency and time should be invested in training over the years. There are many ways to teach dental radiography but the goal is always the same – diagnostic images in as little time as possible. It is advisable to attend lectures and wet labs throughout your years as a technician to learn new tips and tricks or different ways of thinking through positioning. A set of bone skulls should be purchased; these will help with practicing the various angles or a new technique you may have learned.

Full-Mouth Radiographs versus Areas of Concern

A full-mouth radiograph is a set of images that includes all the teeth in the mouth. Full-mouth radiographs are important to establish a baseline and diagnose pathology, especially below the gum line. This is accomplished with 10–12 images for felines and 12 plus images for canines and it is recommended to include lateral views of all four canine teeth. Although these are the minimum number of images, for a large dog it may take significantly more (2–4 times more) to completely image all crowns and roots. Ideally, full-mouth radiographs should be taken annually or at each dental cleaning.

If full-mouth radiographs are not taken at each dental cleaning, radiographs should always be taken of any teeth that are not normal, have evidence of periodontal disease around them, or have changed since the last dental exam. Some of the reasons a tooth should be radiographed, although it is by no means a complete list, are as follows:

- Fractures, abrasion, attrition to teeth
- Displaced, discolored, or mobile teeth
- Missing or supernumerary teeth
- Teeth with periodontal pockets
- Focally increased periodontal disease
- Gingival recession
- Gingival enlargement/oral mass
- Malocclusions
- Maxillary/mandibular bone fractures
- Persistent deciduous teeth
- Nasal discharge
- Facial swelling or draining tracts

Crowns and Roots versus Roots Only

Ideally all crowns and roots should be radiographed for a complete dental set. This provides a record of any crown defects at the time the radiographs are taken. Some may choose to radiograph only the portion of the tooth that cannot be seen with the naked eye, namely, the root. In this case, it is extremely important to include the structures from the marginal gingiva/cementoenamel junction (CEJ)/alveolar crest apically as well as 2–3 mm of surrounding bone as these structures cannot normally be visualized.

Patient Positioning

Dental radiographs can be taken with the patient in any position typically used for dental procedures. Taking radiographs in the position you plan to use to perform your procedures will help minimize the amount of time spent positioning the patient for radiographs alone and then changing their position to perform procedures. Many people learn to take dental radiographs with the patient in sternal recumbency for maxillary radiographs and dorsal recumbency for mandibular radiographs. However, dental radiographs with the patient in lateral recumbency are becoming more commonplace as this seems to be a position used by many veterinarians to perform dental procedures. Another common position is all dorsal recumbency for both dental radiographs and procedures. The positioning of the patient is strictly a veterinarian/technician preference and will not affect the final radiographs. Taking your radiographs with the patient in a new position will likely require practice.

Sensor/Plate/Film Placement within the Oral Cavity

For most of this discussion on positioning and placement of the media, the term "sensor" will be used to mean any of the media (sensor/plate/film) unless otherwise stated. Remember that there are slight differences in which side of each medium faces the teeth. Placing the sensor/plate/film in backward, with the wrong side facing the teeth, will result in a nondiagnostic image, so care should be taken to insert the medium correctly.

Film has a raised dot in one corner and some phosphor plates have a mark in one corner to assist in orienting these media. The raised dot on film is the root of much contention, namely, "Where to place the dot?" Some people always place the raised film dot on the right and some to the front of the mouth. Others prefer to always place the dot on the labial/buccal side of the teeth, regardless of whether this places the dot rostral or distal in the mouth. Pick one method and be consistent in using it. I prefer to place the dot labial/buccal to the teeth to be radiographed because the dot will then never be in the roots of the teeth, potentially obscuring or distorting an important portion of the image (Fig. 6.16). For phosphor plates, follow the manufacturer's recommendation for where to orient any marked corner.

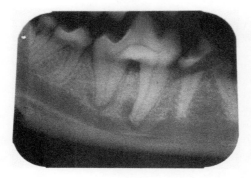

Figure 6.16 Mark from film clip causes difficulty in evaluating tooth root in the upper left. Light leaking into the chairside box caused the defect on the right side.

Sensor placement within the oral cavity is the same regardless of the patient's position and is the same for maxilla and mandible. Most of the sensor should always be inside the pet's mouth with the cable coming out the front of the mouth, not the side. This keeps the tooth/sensor/software orientation and allows the image to display the correct way on your computer screen. Phosphor plates and film obviously do not have a cable. You should be careful to place any identifying markers as instructed earlier.

If you plan to radiograph the entire tooth, have the occlusal tip of the crown near the outer edge of the sensor. This allows you to get the entire crown in the image and, on smaller patients, the entire root plus 2–3 mm of surrounding bone. For larger teeth you will need to move the sensor off the crown for a second radiograph to acquire images of the entire root and surrounding bone.

The sensor can be held in place using gauze, paper towel, foam wedges, or any number of available materials to keep the sensor tight to the teeth, hard palate, or mandible. The sensor should never be held in the mouth by hand, not even with lead gloves on, when taking a radiograph. Phosphor plates and film should never be folded, bent sharply, or creased as this will create distortion of the image and will ruin a phosphor plate. To prevent distortion from bending you may use a wooden tongue depressor behind the film to provide a flat surface (Fig. 6.17).

Incisor crowns should be placed along the short edge of the sensor, near the edge with the cable. The remainder of the sensor is in the mouth along the hard palate or the tongue/floor of the mouth, depending on which incisors are being imaged (see Fig. 6.17).

Canine teeth will require the occlusal tip of the crown to be placed on the sensor's outer corner on the side near the cable for images that include the crown. The rest of the sensor will angle into the mouth along the hard palate. This will give an image of the canine tooth crown and root for smaller teeth. It will give an image of the crown only on larger teeth and a second image of the canine tooth root is needed. Start with the cable edge of the sensor on the hard palate near the mesial aspect of the canine tooth and extending caudally. Some very large teeth may require you to move your sensor further caudally, or in rare cases take a third image.

Premolars and molars will need the occlusal tips of these teeth on the long edge of the sensor with the remaining sensor in the mouth. As with large canine teeth,

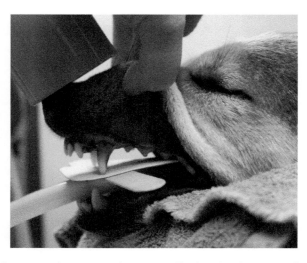

Figure 6.17   Wooden tongue depressor used to prevent film from bending in mouth.

maxillary fourth premolars and mandibular first molars may require more than one radiograph to image both the crown and root.

Tube Head Positioning

There are two common positioning techniques typically used for intraoral images in veterinary dentistry: the parallel technique and the bisecting angle technique. Regardless of the terminology used, all methods use these basic concepts. I will also discuss using the degrees on the tube head scale (scale technique) to assist in positioning as many people find the bisecting angle daunting to use and master. Bisecting angle and parallel techniques refer to the "vertical angle" of the tube head. Tube shift or horizontal tube head direction will also be discussed as needed.

Parallel technique

The parallel technique is the easiest technique to learn. This technique can be used for the mandibular fourth premolar and mandibular molars. The sensor is placed in the mouth parallel to the teeth and mandible to be radiographed. The PID is placed as close to the patient/sensor as possible with the end of the PID parallel to the sensor. The exposure is taken, and the image checked on the computer if using a sensor. If a phosphor plate or film was used, it is removed from the mouth and processed as discussed for each media. Be careful to get your sensor all the way caudally to the last molar in dogs as this tooth can be a challenge to radiograph due to its location. Typically, the sensor should follow the line of the mandible to allow adequate root imaging. No other teeth in either arcade allow the sensor to be placed parallel to the roots (Fig. 6.18).

Bisecting angle technique

The second technique is the bisecting angle, which again, refers to the vertical angulation of the tube head. The hard palate prevents the sensor from being placed

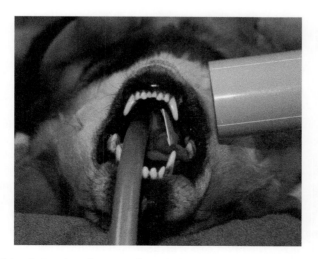

Figure 6.18   Parallel technique in a dog. Note the end of the PID is parallel to the film.

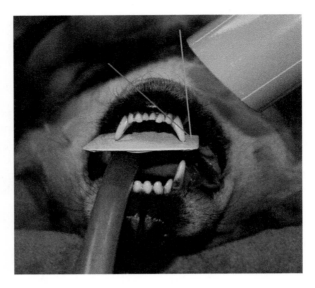

Figure 6.19   Bisecting angle diagram. First note the green line that is the plane of the premolar roots. Next note the plane created by the face of the film. The red line is approximately half way between the two planes. The tube head/PID end is lined up to be parallel to the red line. This is about 45 degrees in this patient.

parallel to the roots of any of the maxillary teeth. The mandibular symphysis prevents the sensor from being placed directly parallel to the mandibular incisors, canine teeth, and first, second, and third premolars. The bisecting angle technique can be challenging to understand but, once mastered, is very useful.

First, determine the plane of the roots of the tooth being radiographed; this is your first plane. Now set your sensor in the mouth as directed in the sensor placement section. The plane created by the face of the sensor is your second plane. An imaginary line halfway between these two planes is your bisecting angle. Now line up the end of the PID parallel to this bisecting angle. A pair of 6 inch cotton swabs, two pens, your fingers, or any number of position aid devices can be used to help you envision the planes of the tooth roots and the sensor as well as the bisecting angle. Do not be afraid to practice, as this is a technique where practice is needed. This method will work with a patient in any position and is very versatile (Fig. 6.19).

Tube Shift or Horizontal Tube Head Direction

This refers to how the tube head/PID lines up with the sensor on the horizontal plane. For most images, the PID should be pointed directly at the sensor without angling rostrally or caudally (oblique). However, for teeth such as the upper fourth premolars, you will need to adjust the tube shift to minimize structures that overlap, namely the two mesial roots. You will do this by aiming your PID/tube head slightly rostrally or caudally. Either direction will help spread out the mesial palatal and mesial buccal roots, so they are not overlapped. Many people struggle to identify the difference between the two mesial roots on their radiographs. If the tube head/PID was angled from the caudal aspect, the middle root is the mesial palatal root. If the tube head/PID was angled from the rostral aspect, the middle root is the mesial buccal root.

CHAPTER 6

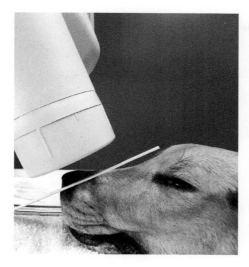

Figure 6.20 Swab creating the proper plane for PID to image maxillary incisors. Note that the end of the PID is parallel to the swab.

When your patient is in lateral recumbency you will need to aim the tube head slightly caudally for imaging the incisors to prevent foreshortening. For maxillary incisors, this correlates nicely with lateral nares slit in dogs. It can be better visualized by placing a cotton swab in this area to form a plane, then have the end of the PID parallel to the swab (Fig. 6.20). This trick works for patients in either lateral or sternal recumbency (see web content: Video 6.1W Dental radiograph positioning).

Scale Technique – Dental Radiographs Simplified

An alternative method to the bisecting angle technique is to use the scale on the tube head where it attaches to the adjustable arm (see Fig. 6.2 at the beginning of this chapter). This scale is available on most machines and correlates to degrees of angulation with "0" having the tube head/PID parallel to the ground/tabletop and "90" having the tube head/PID vertical (straight up and down) or perpendicular to the ground/tabletop. If your dental radiograph machine does not have a scale on it, you can use a protractor to measure the degrees, though some find this tedious.

With this technique, it is important to level the patient's head to minimize variations in the angles used. Leveling the head will be discussed for lateral recumbency and sternal/dorsal recumbency as appropriate to each section for this technique.

Lateral Recumbency and Scale Technique

This section is written assuming the patient is in lateral recumbency. Table 6.1 shows a chart with angles for patients in lateral recumbency for dental radiographs. These angles work for both canines and felines, maxillary teeth and mandibular teeth unless otherwise noted.

To level the head when you are radiographing the maxilla, be sure that the midline of the skull is parallel to the table and the hard palate is vertical (perfectly

Table 6.1   Chart to use for scale technique with patient in lateral recumbency

Lateral	Angle on tube head
Incisors	0 degrees if sensor rests on top of canine teeth
	10 degrees if sensor sits betwen the maxillary canine teeth – this is not needed for mandibular incisors
Canines – lateral image	25 degrees from lateral side
Premolars	
All maxillary premolars	45 degrees for canines 108/208 Slight oblique
1st–3rd mandibular premolars	55 degrees for felines for 108/208 Slight oblique
Maxillary molars	45 degrees from lateral side
Mandibular canine ventrodorsal view	0 degrees from under mandible
Mandibular premolar 4 and molars	Parallel technique – PID edge parallel to sensor

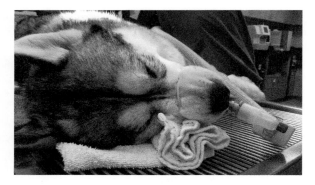

Figure 6.21   Patient with head leveled for maxillary radiographs. Note the wash cloth supporting the muzzle.

straight up and down). This will require you to support the muzzle and be sure the head is not rolled ventrally (Fig. 6.21).

For mandibular imaging, make sure that the mandible being radiographed is parallel to the tabletop. This will require you to raise the chin and roll your patient's head slightly toward the dorsal aspect (Fig. 6.22).

These two head-leveling positions will likely require you to place some small towels, wash cloths, or other positioning aids under the muzzle/skull to help maintain your level planes. This will be important in the early phases of learning to take dental radiographs with this technique. As you become more proficient, you will likely develop the skills to compensate for the changes in degrees encountered by not leveling the head.

Once leveled, you are ready to take radiographs. As you will see in the chart in Table 6.1, the incisors will generally use "0" degrees on the tube head. This means

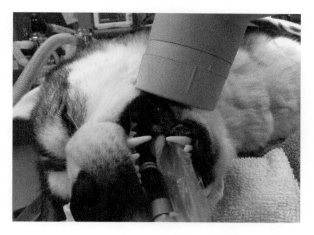

Figure 6.22   Patient's head has the mandible level with table top. Note the wash cloth supporting the mandible.

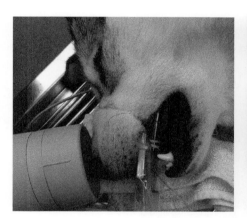
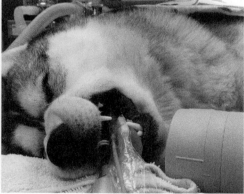

Figure 6.23   Left: Sensor and PID placement for maxillary incisors. Note the end of the PID is parallel to the imaginary line at the lateral nares slit. Scale is set at 0 degrees. Remember that 10 degrees may be needed for the lateral incisor. Right: Sensor and PID placement for mandibular incisors. Scale is at 0 degrees. Note the slight caudal aim of the PID/tube head to prevent foreshortening of the incisor image.

the tube head is parallel to your tabletop. As you move caudally, taking radiographs, you will notice that the degrees gradually become steeper (that is, the number on the tube head becomes larger). In general, incisors are taken at "0" degrees (see exception), canine teeth at "25" degrees for both maxilla and mandible. All maxillary premolars/molars and the mandibular first/second/third premolars are taken at "45" degrees (Figs. 6.23–6.28). (Note: The slight tilt of the sensor as it goes from the tooth crown to the oral structures usually does not cause problems in this author's experience. However, if you wish, you may place some gauze between the sensor and the palate to allow the sensor to lie perfectly parallel to the hard palate.)

Mandibular fourth premolars and molars are taken using the parallel technique. No tube head angles are used.

Horizontal tube shift is as discussed earlier.

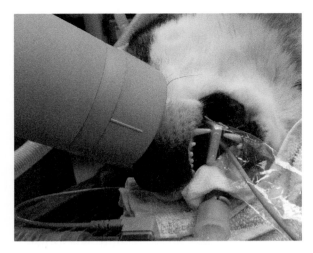

Figure 6.24 PID placement for maxillary canine image. Scale is set at 25 degrees. Remember that on a large dog like this you will likely need a second image of the root.

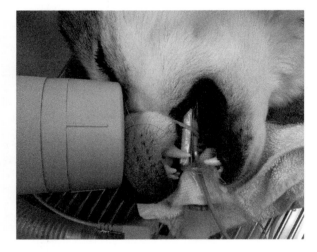

Figure 6.25 Sensor placement and PID placement for canine tooth root. Scale is set at 25 degrees.

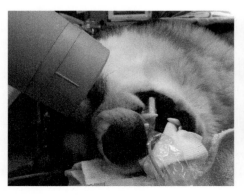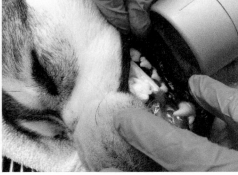

Figure 6.26 Left: Sensor and PID placement for premolars. Scale is set at 45 degrees. Right: Sensor and PID placement for mandibular premolars. Scale is set at 45 degrees.

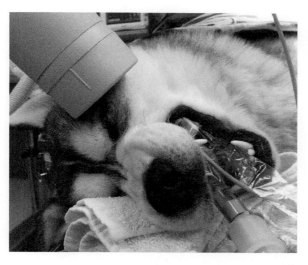

Figure 6.27   Sensor and PID placement for maxillary fourth premolar. Note the PID is pointed slightly caudal to rostral. Scale is still set at 45 degrees.

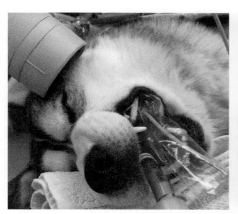 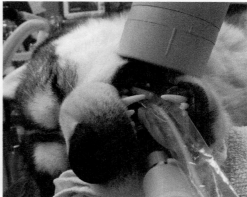

Figure 6.28   Left: Sensor and PID placement for maxillary molars. Scale is still set at 45 degrees. The sensor may need to be angled into the mouth slightly to get around the ramus of the mandible. Right: Sensor and PID placement for mandibular molars. Note the sensor is parallel to the mandible and the PID end is parallel to the sensor.

There are two exceptions to the above techniques, but they are generally easy to adjust for:

■ **Maxillary third incisors:** If the sensor sits on top of both maxillary canine teeth crowns, use "0" to image all six incisors. However, if the sensor falls between the canine teeth, as with medium to large dogs, you will likely need to take a couple of images of the incisors. The first image will be of the four central incisors and taken at "0" degrees. The maxillary third incisor will be too close to the edge of the sensor to be completely imaged. You will move the sensor as close to the canine tooth as possible and adjust your tube head angle to "10" degrees. Most of the time, you will get the third incisor with this change in degrees. Some technicians will opt to take this image on large dogs to radiograph the three incisors

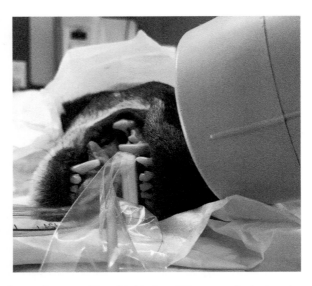

Figure 6.29   Lateral exception – maxillary third incisor. PID same as for incisors but with scale at 10 degrees instead of 0.

on the right side. They will repeat this radiograph for the three incisors on the left side when the patient is repositioned. They will forego the radiograph of the four central maxillary incisors as they will already be imaged. This is acceptable in most cases, although you should refer to your veterinarian for their preference (Fig. 6.29).

■ **Feline maxillary fourth premolars:** Because of their zygomatic arch, you will likely need to use "55" degrees instead of "45" degrees to image this tooth. The "45" degrees will work well for the maxillary second and third premolars in the feline patient, just not the fourth premolar. On rare occasions, you may need to use an even steeper angle. This will reflect the zygomatic arch dorsally. Some overlap of the zygomatic arch on the tooth roots is acceptable if the periodontal ligament can be seen around the entire root, although you should refer to your veterinarian for their preference.

Using the scale technique, with your patient in lateral recumbency, if you get foreshortening, increase your vertical angle. If you encounter elongation, decrease your vertical angle. In general, an adjustment of 5–8 degrees for small patients and 10–12 degrees for larger patients is enough to change the image.

Sternal/Dorsal Recumbency and Scale Technique

This section assumes the patient is in sternal recumbency for maxillary images and dorsal recumbency for mandibular images. Table 6.2 shows a chart with angles for patients in sternal/dorsal recumbency. Again, the angles work for both felines and canines, maxillary or mandibular teeth.

As before, you will need to level the patient's head. For maxillary teeth, be sure the hard palate is parallel to your tabletop or level from front to back and side to side.

Table 6.2   Chart to use for scale technique with patient in sternal/dorsal recumbency

Sternal/dorsal	Angle on tube head
Incisors	55 degrees or follow the line created by the lateral nares slit
	Slightly oblique if sensor sits between the maxillary canine teeth – this is not needed for mandibular incisors
Canines – lateral image	65 degrees from lateral side
Premolars	
All maxillary premolars with patient in sternal recumbency	45 degrees for canine patients for 108/208 Slight oblique
1st–3rd mandibular premolars with patient in dorsal recumbency	35 degrees for felines for 108/208 Slight oblique
Maxillary molars	45 degrees both canine and feline patients
Mandibular canine ventrodorsal view	PID end will be parallel to the sensor
Mandibular premolar 4 and molars	Parallel technique – PID edge parallel to sensor

Tipping of the head can cause issues using the numbers on the tube head. For mandibular teeth, be sure to level the mandibles both front to back and side to side.

As with the lateral technique, both positions will likely require you to place some small towels, wash cloths, or other positioning aids under the muzzle or neck to help maintain your level planes. Again, this will be important in the early phases of your learning to take dental radiographs with this technique. As you become more proficient, you will likely develop the skills to compensate for the changes in degrees encountered by not leveling the head.

Once leveled, you are ready to check the chart in Table 6.2 for sternal/dorsal recumbency. For the incisors, you will use 55 degrees though this will vary depending on skull/muzzle shape. Again, the lateral nares slit in dogs can be helpful for imaging the maxillary incisor. If you place a cotton swab in this area to form a plane, you can line up your PID end parallel to the swab. This almost always gives the proper angulation for imaging the maxillary incisors.

Canine teeth, both maxilla and mandible, use 65 degrees. Maxillary premolars/ molars and mandibular first, second, and third premolars use 45 degrees. You will notice that with sternal/dorsal recumbency your tube head angles will decrease as you move caudally (Figs. 6.30–6.35).

Mandibular incisors, canine teeth, and premolars are imaged using these degrees with your patient in dorsal recumbency and the mandibles leveled. Parallel technique will be used for the remaining mandibular teeth – no tube head numbers are used.

Using this technique with your patient in sternal or dorsal recumbency, foreshortening errors will require you to decrease your angle to correct the problem; elongation errors will require you to increase your angle to correct it.

Tube shift is the same as discussed earlier.

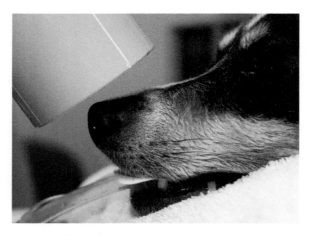

Figure 6.30   Sensor and PID placement for patients in sternal recumbency. Note the PID is parallel to the lateral nares slit. It correlates loosely with 55 degrees for most patients.

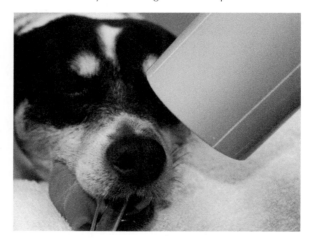

Figure 6.31   Sensor PID placement for canine tooth. Scale is set at 25 degrees. Remember that in larger patients you will need a second radiograph of the root.

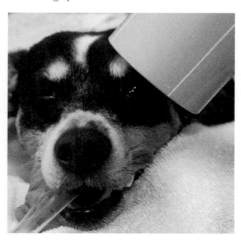

Figure 6.32   Sensor and PID placement for premolars. Scale is at 45 degrees for the remaining maxillary teeth.

CHAPTER 6

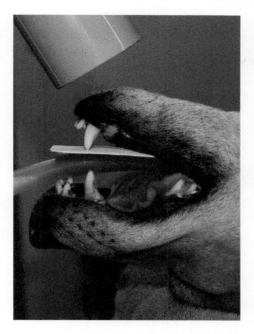

Figure 6.33 Patient in dorsal recumbency. Sensor and PID placement. Scale is set at 55 degrees.

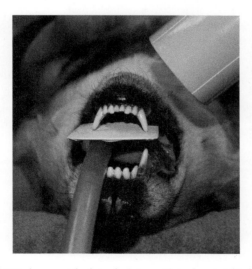

Figure 6.34 Sensor and PID placement for lateral canine with scale set at 25 degrees. Sensor and PID placement will be similar for premolars 1–3 with the scale set at 45.

Again, there are a few exceptions and you will have to adjust for the same teeth:

- **Maxillary third incisor:** This tooth will still be close to the edge of the sensor on your larger patients where the sensor sits between to maxillary canine teeth. It will require adjustment of the tube shift since your patient is in sternal recumbency. Simply oblique your angle slightly, that is, move your tube head from pointing ventrocaudal at the incisors to being slightly off to the side (oblique). You will still use 55 degrees, and this will project the image onto the sensor. Some

CHAPTER 6

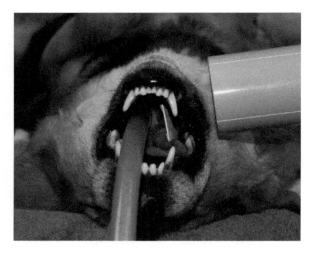

Figure 6.35   Sensor and PID placement for parallel technique for mandibular P4 and molars. There is no scale degree as the PID end should be parallel to your sensor as shown here with dental film.

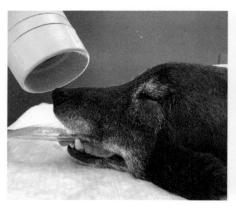 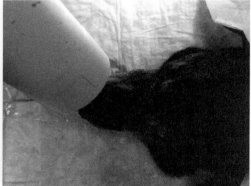

Figure 6.36   Exception maxillary third incisor in sternal. Line the PID up for a regular incisor image then shift the PID slightly around the nose to the lateral side (only about a quarter of the way).

technicians opt to take this image on large dogs and radiograph the three incisors on the right side. They will repeat this radiograph for the three incisors on the left side and will forego the radiograph of the four central maxillary incisors as they will already be imaged. This is acceptable in most cases although you should refer to your veterinarian for their preference (Fig. 6.36).

■ **Feline upper fourth premolars:** These will likely require you to use 35 degrees to avoid the zygomatic arch. Some felines may require an even shorter angle. This will reflect the zygomatic arch dorsally. Some overlap on the zygomatic arch on the tooth roots is acceptable if the periodontal ligament can be seen around the entire root.

Dorsal Only Recumbency

Some clinics perform dental procedures with the patient in dorsal recumbency. Taking radiographs in this position is done using a combination of the techniques described earlier.

Some clinics take the preliminary maxillary radiographs right after intubation as the patient is usually in sternal recumbency. Then they reposition the patient in dorsal recumbency to take mandibular radiographs. Thus, they follow the techniques for sternal/dorsal positions.

Other clinics will position the patient in dorsal recumbency and take all their mandibular radiographs, then turn the patient's head to each side in turn to perform the left and right maxillary radiographs. This may require shifting the patient's body slightly to one side or the other but in general still allows the monitoring equipment and fluid line to remain attached. You can use any of the described methods for taking the mandibular radiographs. However, when taking the maxillary radiographs in this manner, leveling the head (as described for using the tube head scale) is challenging. Thus, bisecting angle is generally the surest way to get diagnostic images quickly.

Note that the numbers in these charts are just a starting point. Because there are so many different breeds and mixed breeds, there are many different skull shapes, and these affect the angles used. These angles will work in most cases.

It is very important to remove as many variables as possible. The patient's skull should always be in the same position each time. Level the head before you start, or the degrees will not work consistently.

Care and Storage of Images

The care and correct storage of all dental radiographic images are extremely important. Images are part of the legal medical record for each patient and must be handled as such. They are a record of pathology prior to dental treatment and your record of successful treatment afterward. Pre- and postextraction radiographs are required for all extractions as well as any dental treatment that changes teeth or bone structures.

Identification of digital images is built into most software as it requires you to begin a new patient and thus provide identification of the image set. Owner's name, patient name, and date are the minimum requirements for identification. If that patient has previous dental radiographs in the system, you will start a new date for the new image set under the preexisting patient. Some software will allow minimal input to start taking images. If this is the case, it is imperative that you go back afterward and label the image set. Additional information can usually be entered to help identify each patient, such as the practice management software client/pet ID number. Depending on the computer software used, some allow images to be downloaded into the practice management software for each individual pet.

All digital dental radiographs should be backed up or copied to an additional storage location. Backups and/or hard copies are important with digital systems to preserve the images should a computer malfunction. Digital file sizes can be large and may require additional computer hard drive space on the primary or acquisition computer or on another system designed for backing up files. As we move into the digital age, backup options are numerous, from small, external hard drives to cloud-based services. Be sure your clinic has these valuable files protected.

Identification of standard film is important and can be a challenge due to their small size. Each individual series of images should be identified with client name, patient name, and the date taken. Be sure films are completely dry before storing to prevent them from sticking to each other or the envelopes. A common method of identification

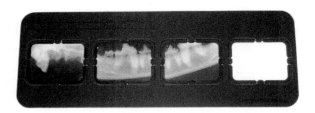

Figure 6.37   Films mounted in a film mount. Be sure to orient the films the correct way for convenient viewing.

is to place the films in film mounts. Film mounts are paperboard or plastic frames with holes for each film and tabs to clip in the films (Fig. 6.37). As another option, radiographic numbers can be placed on the films prior to exposure with the numbers and patient information recorded in a radiology log.[5-7] Films can also be labeled with a permanent marker in a way that does not affect the area of interest, though this can be difficult due to their size. Once numbered or placed in mounts, films should be placed in envelopes and stored either with each patient's record or in a separate radiograph file. Film should be stored in a cool, dry location as moisture can soften the emulsion and cause films to stick together, even after proper processing.

Anatomy on the Dental Radiograph[5]

Interpretation of the radiographic image is as important as creating a high-quality image. It is recommended that you take full-mouth radiographs for comparison of the right to left arcades and from one dental procedure to the next. Solid knowledge of anatomical structures and their location is beneficial to determine normal from abnormal. Although not all anatomical features can be seen on every radiograph, being familiar with them allows accurate identification and interpretation when seen. Keep in mind that there is some variation that can still be considered normal and it sometimes depends on the angle when taking the image or age, breed, and species of the animal.

Intraoral images should be viewed in labial presentation. Please refer to the discussion about labial presentation under the section "Reading the Dental Radiographic Image" in "Dental Radiographic Image Media and Capture". As stated in that text, it is important to be able to identify individual teeth as well as the arcades.

Learning what is normal is a large part of identifying what is abnormal. Once your image is correctly oriented, assess the entire film for the quality of exposure and developing, and whether the tooth in question, both crown and root, appear in your radiograph. The radiograph should have a clear image without blurring, splotching, or fogging. All roots should be visible with a minimum of 2–3 mm visible beyond the apices. This allows you to view the full periodontal ligament, lamina dura, and some of the alveolar bone.

Next look at all the structures in the view. It is easy to get sidetracked or make quick assessments if there is an obvious defect; however, you do not want to miss the less obvious issues either. Check out the bony tissue present; does it appear normal and consistent? Do you have an adequate amount of structure visible to assess it? Your radiograph should extend well beyond the roots of the teeth in question. Remember the minimum 2–3 mm rule.

Then start on the left and move to the right; look at each tooth – does the dentin and pulp cavity match its neighbors, is the periodontal ligament visible all the way around the root, is the alveolar bone at the proper height (any signs of vertical or horizontal bone loss), any resorption or periapical lucency? Perform these steps with each tooth as you move to the right.

Keep in mind that radiolucent objects will appear black and radiodense objects are white; thus air is black, and bone/tooth will appear white or shades of gray. Starting with the crown of the tooth, the enamel is often difficult to differentiate on the crown of the tooth, but a white line may be seen at the edge of the crown. Dentin is seen as medium density and encompasses most of the tooth, both crown and root, of the typical adult tooth. The pulp cavity is the central, more radiolucent space of the tooth and occurs in both the crown and the root. If the animal is younger, the dentin will be a narrower line between the enamel and the pulp cavity and the pulp cavity will be quite wide. As animals age, the pulp cavity goes from very wide with a narrow line of dentin, to a narrow pulp cavity and a wide area of dentin. The cementum on the root of the tooth is ill-defined in radiographs and will be outlined by a radiolucent (black) line, the periodontal ligament. The lamina dura is the thin, very radiodense line in the alveolar bone that forms the tooth socket. Beyond that is the cortical bone that forms the jaw and alveolar crest. Be aware that the various foramina on the jaw can appear as lesions or radiolucent spots in the jaw. Knowing where these are located is very beneficial to interpretation (Fig. 6.38).

Common radiographic pathology to learn to identify includes missing or unerupted teeth, horizontal and vertical bone loss, endodontic lesions, abnormal root structure, retained tooth roots, tooth resorption, and fractures to the roots or bone below the gum line. This is by no means a complete list of the pathology that may be seen but it is a good start to identifying problems seen with radiographs.

Missing and unerupted teeth are obvious. A missing tooth is one that is not visible in the mouth, and on the radiograph is also not present within the bone. An unerupted tooth is not visible in the mouth but can be seen on the radiograph below the gingiva and possibly impacted (prevented from erupting by another structure). Be sure you have a radiograph that goes to the ventral border of the mandible or to the maxillary sinuses and at least one tooth beyond the normal area for the missing tooth. Remember that the tooth may be in an abnormal position if unerupted.

There are several problems to look for when analyzing radiographs for periodontal disease. Periodontal bone loss will be either horizontal or vertical. Normal bone

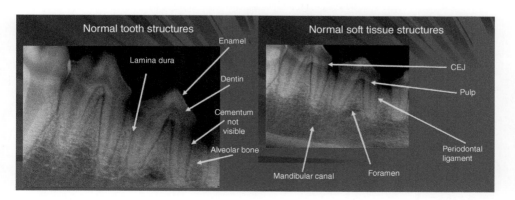

Figure 6.38   Normal radiographic structures.

should reach the CEJ and fill the furcation of a tooth. Horizontal bone loss is seen as bone receding from the CEJ and/or furcation of the tooth apically in a horizontal line across the tooth. Vertical bone loss is seen as bone loss that follows one or more roots apically.

Endodontic disease may not be obvious until you take a radiograph. Endodontic disease is exhibited in several ways on radiographs. It may be a pulp canal that is different in size in the affected tooth than other teeth in the same mouth. Compare the tooth in question to the neighboring teeth and the identical tooth on the other side of the mouth. Is the canal similar in size? If not, the tooth will warrant further evaluation. You may see periapical lucency as a darker gray, radiolucent bubble or line around the apex of one or more roots. This bubble can vary in size or shape and the foramen can mimic periapical lucency, so be cautious and know your anatomy. Sometimes these changes can be very subtle, showing only a slight widening of the periodontal ligament space or a disruption of the lamina dura (Fig. 6.39).

Root abnormalities vary from root tips that curve in unusual directions to extra roots. This is very important information when planning extractions as the procedure may need to be adjusted to accommodate an extra root or a tip that is curved in an unusual fashion. Fractures of the roots will appear as a solid dark gray line across the root. If the fracture involves bone, the gray line will appear in the bone as well. Retained roots will appear as white densities in the bone subgingival to where a tooth crown is missing. They usually have a periodontal ligament visible around them though not always.

Tooth resorption can vary. Teeth with tooth resorption will have an abnormal gray area in the crown and/or root. The tooth may appear to have a large piece missing from it or have a moth-eaten appearance. The roots can have a normal periodontal ligament space with only the crown affected or the periodontal ligament can be almost nonexistent with the root and surrounding bone hard to differentiate. These teeth are in the process of ankylosis.

Learning radiographic anatomy and recognizing pathology can be a challenging part of taking dental radiographs. With a bit of practice, this skill will expedite the diagnosis of several treatable diseases in the oral cavity.

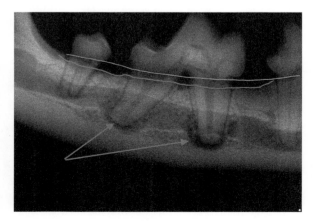

Figure 6.39 Note the periapical lucency on both roots of the mandibular first molar. (blue arrows). Also note the abnormal roots on the mandibular second molar. There is visible horizontal bone loss on both teeth (red line). The green line indicates normal bone height.

Troubleshooting

Troubleshooting with digital images is minimal in most cases. The most common errors are positioning, cone cutting, and over- or underexposure. As earlier, the word "sensor" is used here to mean any of the dental media.

Elongation and foreshortening were briefly discussed at the end of each section on lateral/sternal/dorsal recumbency as these positions each require their own corrections. Elongation can accentuate pathology and make vertical and horizontal bone loss appear worse or deeper along the tooth root. Foreshortening can minimize the appearance of bone loss and even hide pathology, especially within the furcation area of a tooth. Remember that the tooth on the radiograph should look like the tooth in the mouth, with a proper crown-to-root ratio (Fig. 6.40).

Cone cutting results in not having the PID or tube head centered over the sensor. The final image will have a sharp, white, curved line on one side of the image. While not desirable, if it does not cut off structures of interest, nothing needs to be done. However, as in most cases, if it cuts off structure that needs to be examined, a retake is needed. To correct, move the PID in the direction of the missing or whited out image. Be sure the PID is centered over the sensor. Some people will move the PID further from the sensor/patient, however, this allows the radiation to spread out further. Although it may resolve the cone cutting, it can reduce the amount of radiation that contacts the sensor, affecting the image quality and resulting in more

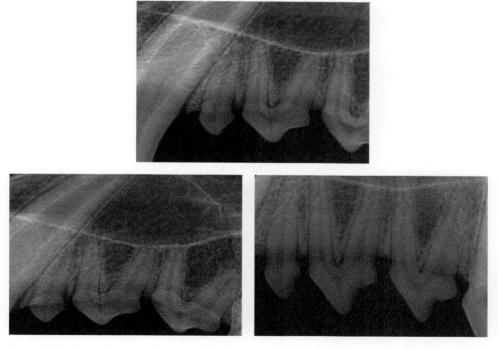

Figure 6.40 Elongation versus foreshortening. The top image has correct angulation. The lower left shows foreshortening, note the crown overlapping the furcation, making evaluation challenging. The lower right image show elongation. Tooth roots are stretched, creating horizontal bone loss that does not truly exist. Correct this by changing your vertical angulation.

radiation scatter. A more accurate way of correcting this error is to center your PID over your sensor (Fig. 6.41).

Overexposure is caused by too much radiation being generated and contacting the sensor. It generally causes an image that is too dark or burned out and lacks areas of white where the bone is dense. Crowns of teeth that are present in the mouth may appear missing; the alveolar crest and other thin structures may not be visible on the radiograph. To correct this, decrease the time setting on the control panel. This will reduce the amount of radiation and is the simplest way to correct the problem.

Underexposure is caused by not enough radiation contacting the sensor. It generally causes an image that is too light, has too much white, or even has a hazy appearance. There is usually a lack of black areas where no tissue is present. These areas may be various shades of gray but lack true black. These can cause pathology to be missed as the white haze may hide or fail to show areas of pathology. To correct this, increase the time setting on the control panel. This will increase the amount of radiation sent to the sensor, giving more shades of gray and areas of true black (Fig. 6.42).

Positioning errors are the most common errors by far. Careful placement of the sensor, attention to tube head angle and, if using the tube head scale technique, levelness of the head, all play a part in positioning. Correct these first. Then, if the oral

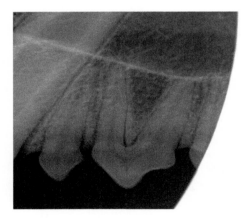

Figure 6.41 Cone cutting. Notice how cone cutting prevents viewing the distal third premolar. Correct this by centering the PID over the sensor. In this case, you would move your PID caudally.

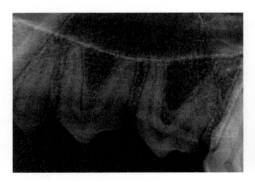 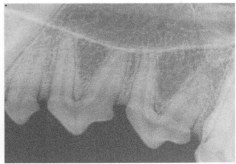

Figure 6.42 Overexposure and underexposure can make reading your radiographs challenging. Correct it by adjusting the time on the control panel.

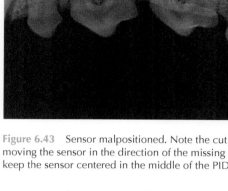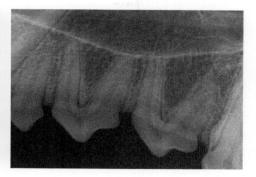

Figure 6.43   Sensor malpositioned. Note the cut off tooth roots on the left image. Correct this by moving the sensor in the direction of the missing structure. Be sure to reposition the PID if needed to keep the sensor centered in the middle of the PID.

structure of interest is off the edge of the sensor, move the sensor in the direction of the missed structure. Always recenter the PID over the sensor (Fig. 6.43).

Remember that there is always more to learn about positioning and practice is the key!

Advanced Imaging

Computed tomography (CT) uses radiation and takes multiple radiographs in thin slices to produce a digital image that can be reconstructed to create a three-dimensional (3D) image.[7] It is generally accepted that CT is best for bone imaging and is becoming more commonplace for imaging prior to jaw fracture repair, surgical procedures to determine the extent of neoplasia involvement, surgical reconstruction and temporomandibular joint (TMJ) dysfunction treatment. Using these images, a 3D printer can create a full-scale model of the structure to allow additional options for preplanning of difficult procedures. Patients require heavy sedation or general anesthesia and these units can require large amounts of space, special permits, and room modifications. They still are not widely available, and images generally need to be evaluated by a radiologist (Fig. 6.44).

Cone beam computed tomography (CBCT) is rapidly gaining favor as a modality that may be useful in veterinary dentistry. Although it uses radiation as a standard CT, some feel it can be less, although it depends largely on the system and the size of the area imaged. It is superior to dental radiographs and standard CT in many cases due to the exceedingly high resolution, though the resolution may be affected by software choice. It appears that software may be very important in determining image quality.[5] CBCT can be used to identify small areas of bone loss on failed endodontic therapy (that appears successful on radiographs), periodontal disease, and allows imaging of feline maxillary teeth without overlapping structures such as the zygomatic arch. CBCT excels for imaging small areas and small structures.

In addition, CBCT units tend to have a smaller footprint than standard CT units, can be used within a dental suite, and allow imaging without moving the patient. Disadvantages are that they still use more radiation than dental radiographs, image resolution is affected by software choice and thus may not be as good as desired, and

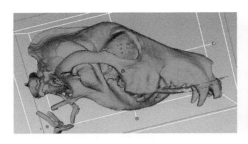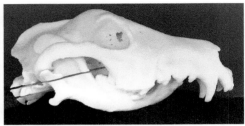

Figure 6.44   Three-dimensional computed tomography image and printed model.

the cost and size of the units in addition to imaging only small areas. They may not be sufficient for larger areas such as neoplasia or fractures.[5]

Magnetic resonance imaging (MRI) uses magnetic fields and a radio signal to create digital images.[8] This helps limit the amount of radiation clinic staff and patients are exposed to for procedures. The MRI produces images in small slices much like a CT. These can then be digitally reconstructed to give a 3D look to the tissues imaged as well as to allow 3D printing. In the past, it was generally thought that MRI was superior for soft tissue but not always the best for bone imaging. This is changing as technology advances and bone resolution improves.[8] Availability and cost remain the common limiting factors for using MRI, as does the need for heavy sedation or general anesthesia. MRI units require special rooms, permits, large amounts of space, highly trained staff, and a radiologist to interpret images. Given the availability of technologies such as dental radiographs, CBCT, and standard CT, it is unlike that MRI will be routinely used for dental imaging in the near future.

See Appendix 6 for dental radiograph template.

References

1. Gorrel, C, Derbyshire, S. 2005. *Veterinary Dentistry for the Nurse and Technician* (ed. M Seager). Philadelphia, PA: Elsevier.
2. Bellows, J. 1999. *The Practice of Veterinary Dentistry*. Ames, IA: Iowa State Press.
3. Holmstrom, SE, Bellows, J, Juriga, S, Knutson, K, Niemiec, BA, Perrone, J. 2013. AAHA dental care guidelines for dogs and cats. *Journal of the American Animal Hospital Association* 49:75–82.
4. Basset, J, McCurnin, D. 2010. *McCurnin's Clinical Textbook for Veterinary Technicians* (ed. T Merchant). St. Louis, MO: Saunders Elsevier.
5. Niemiec, BA, Gawor, J, Jekl, V. 2018. *Practical Veterinary Dental Radiography*. Boca Raton, FL: CRC Press.
6. Holmstrom, S. 2000. *Veterinary Dentistry for the Technician and Office Staff*. Philadelphia, PA: WB Saunders.
7. Feeney, DA, Fletcher, TF, Hardy, RM. 1991. *Atlas of Correlative Imaging Anatomy of the Normal Dog*. Philadelphia, PA: WB Saunders.
8. Dennis, R. 1993. Magnetic resonance imaging and its application to veterinary medicine. *Veterinary International* 6:3–10.

Common Dental Conditions and Treatments

7

Jeanne R. Perrone, MS, CVT, VTS (Dentistry), Sara Sharp, CVT, VTS (Dentistry), and Patricia A. March, RVT, VTS (Dentistry)

Learning Objectives

- Define periodontal disease
- Describe the pathogenesis or development of periodontal disease
- Identify the clinical signs of periodontal disease found during the oral exam
- Demonstrate how dental radiographs are used to diagnose and assess the severity of periodontal disease
- Identify the commonly used treatments and therapies for periodontal disease
- Describe the anatomy of the pulp
- Discuss the indications for endodontic therapy
- Discuss what to look for during an endodontic examination
- Discuss the different types of endodontic treatments
- Describe the steps involved for each type of endodontic therapy
- Identify common oral malocclusions
- Explain the complications that each type of oral malocclusion can cause
- Present the current treatment for the each type of malocclusion
- Explain how the veterinary technician assists the veterinarian with oral surgery
- Describe the different types of jaw fractures
- Identify the various treatment options for jaw fracture management
- Compile postoperative patient care instructions for the client/pet owner
- Describe common oral tumors, both benign and malignant
- Discuss the current modalities of treatments for various oral tumors
- Describe the correct handling and processing of biopsy samples

Small Animal Dental Procedures for Veterinary Technicians and Nurses, Second Edition.
Edited by Jeanne R. Perrone.
© 2021 John Wiley & Sons, Inc. Published 2021 by John Wiley & Sons, Inc.

Introduction

This chapter deals with dental conditions that will come through the general practice – periodontal disease, endodontic disease, malocclusion, jaw fractures, and oral tumors. Some of these cases, once diagnosed in the general practice, may require the help of a board-certified veterinary dentist or another specialist.

So if some of these cases may end up with a veterinary dentist, or another specialist, why does the technician working in the general practice need to be familiar with these conditions? The general practice is the front line that begins the diagnostic and treatment process. In the case of a jaw fracture, it stabilizes the patient before the dental treatment. The technician is, in some cases, responsible for keeping the owner informed of the patient's status and treatment options. If the technician understands the disease process and the treatment options, they are better able to serve both the veterinarian and the client.

The learning objectives for each section are stated at the beginning of this chapter.

Periodontal Disease

Jeanne R. Perrone, MS, CVT, VTS (Dentistry)

What is Periodontal Disease?

Periodontal disease is a bacterial inflammation of the periodontium or periodontal tissues. It is the most common oral condition found in dogs and a common condition in cats.[1,2] The periodontal tissues are those structures that hold the tooth in the mouth. Those structures, known as the periodontium, include the gingiva, the periodontal ligament, and the alveolar bone.[1]

Pathogenesis of Periodontal Disease

Pellicle

The oral cavity is a consistently moist environment. The pellicle is a thin film consisting of salivary proteins and glycoproteins. It protects and lubricates. Pellicle deposition occurs immediately after a dental cleaning. As the pellicle ages, it gives a surface to which the oral bacteria can adhere.[1]

Dental Plaque

As bacteria colonize the pellicle, a biofilm forms on the inert surfaces of the tooth, namely the crown; this becomes mature plaque. It is difficult to see but can be visualized using a plaque-disclosing solution. The biofilm thickens as the aerobic bacteria consume oxygen and multiply, making the environment more suitable for anaerobic bacteria. An important thing to remember here is that dental plaque is not a disease, but is the cause of periodontal disease. Plaque that is allowed to accumulate will result in gingivitis.[1]

Dental Calculus

Dog and cat mouths, unlike human mouths, are slightly alkaline, an environment in which calcium salts are more likely to be deposited. Calcium carbonate and calcium phosphate salts are found in the salivary fluid. These calcium products crystallize on the surface of the teeth and mineralize the soft plaque.[1] The formation of dental calculus takes 2–3 days. The deep crevices along the surface of the calculus promote further growth of anaerobic bacteria because oxygen is low to unavailable.[1] Calculus cannot be removed except by mechanical action (hand or power scaling).

Gingivitis

Plaque extends subgingivally, and the mixture of bacteria and cell degradation products become destructive on the periodontal soft tissues, leading to inflammation and gingivitis.[2] Sulcus depths are usually normal. Gingivitis is considered reversible, meaning that once the bacteria-laden dental plaque is removed, the inflammation disappears. Not all sites with gingivitis proceed to periodontitis. Gingivitis can become more severe in patients with local or systemic conditions[1] (Fig. 7.1).

Periodontitis

Periodontitis is the inflammatory destruction of the epithelial barrier that protects the tooth's support structure. The tooth support structures are the gingiva, cementum, periodontal ligament, and the alveolar bone. Bacteria can break through the epithelial barrier if the patient is unable to launch an effective immune response.[1,3] As the bacteria moves deeper into the periodontal tissues, the bacteria run out of oxygen and become more destructive. The epithelial barrier breaks down, and the gingiva separates or shrinks away from the alveolar bone, causing a periodontal

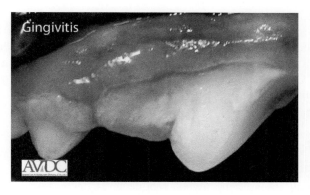

Figure 7.1 Photograph of a maxillary fourth premolar (108) with gingivitis. Note the red line at the gingival margin (Copyright AVDC, used with permission).

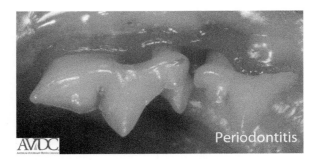

Figure 7.2   Photograph of a maxillary third and fourth premolar (107, 108) with periodontitis. Note the gingival recession, the marked inflammation, and the furcation exposure (Copyright AVDC, used with permission).

pocket or gingival recession. As the bacteria move toward the root, the periodontal ligament and the alveolar bone are destroyed. As more of these support structures are affected, tooth mobility will be seen (Fig. 7.2).

Pathogenic bacteria cause the body to activate immune and nonimmune reactions that are responsible for tissue damage. It is the host response to plaque bacteria and not the virulence of the bacteria that causes the tissue damage. So, all dogs and cats will develop plaque, but not all that plaque will develop into periodontitis.[1]

Clinical Signs

Halitosis or bad breath is the owner complaint when the patient is brought in for an oral exam. When assessing the patient for periodontal disease, part of the examination occurs with the owner present, and the rest of the exam is done under anesthesia.

In the exam room, the whole mouth is given a subjective generalized assessment. At this point, you can classify the severity of the periodontal disease using either the standard periodontal classification disease provided by the American Veterinary Dental College (AVDC) or a classification system used by the veterinary hospital (Table 7.1).

Common clinical signs of periodontal disease are gingival inflammation, gingival recession, periodontal pockets, furcation, and root exposure, presence of purulent discharge, draining tracts, and calculus. The patient may show discomfort when touched around the mouth or when chewing food (Table 7.1).

In most patients, periodontal disease is a preventable condition if dental education, examination and treatment are provided expediently. According to the 2019 AAHA Dental Guidelines, prevention of periodontal disease begins at the first puppy or kitten visit. Oral assessment parameters can be instituted at certain stages of the pediatric examination (Table 7.2).

Radiographic Signs

With periodontal disease, the alveolar bone level decreases as the inflammation moves apically and bone is resorbed.

Table 7.1 Stages of periodontal disease and their treatment options

Classification	Stage	Abbreviation	Gum health	Radiographic changes	Treatment
Normal	Stage 0	PD0	No gingival inflammation	No change to alveolar height or architecture	Prophylactic dental cleaning
Gingivitis	Stage I	PD1	Mild gingival inflammation	No change to alveolar height or architecture	Dental cleaning; subgingival cleaning; home care
Early periodontitis	Stage II	PD2	Gingival Inflammation and swelling; bleeding on probing; 25% attachment loss or stage 1 furcation involvement	Loss of periodontal attachment <25%	All of the above; with or without closed curettage; perioceutics
Moderate periodontitis	Stage III	PD3	Gingival inflammation and swelling; bleeding on probing; gum recession or hyperplasia; 25–50% attachment loss; stage 2 furcation involvement; M1 mobility possible	10–30% loss of bone support	All of the above; flap surgery and/or extractions
Advanced periodontitis	Stage IV	PD4	Gingival inflammation and swelling, bleeding on probing; recession or hyperplasia; >50% attachment loss; pocket depth >5 mm; stage 3 furcation exposure; M2–3 mobility	Over 30% bone loss	All of the above; placement of bone grafting materials if needed; extractions if support loss is >50%

Table 7.2 Assessment parameters using the age of the patient

- Using a life stage approach to evaluate oral hygiene is highly recommended
- From birth to 9 months of age, evaluate the patient for problems related to deciduous teeth, missing or extra teeth, and oral swellings
- From the age of 5 months to 2 years, evaluate for developmental anomalies, permanent dentition, and the accumulation of plaque and calculus
- Toy and small-breed dogs can start showing signs of periodontal disease as early as 9 months
- After 2 years of age, all dogs and cats should be checked for signs of periodontal disease and evaluated for the adequacy of home care

Source: Bellows, JB. 2019. 2019 AAHA dental care guidelines for dogs and cats. *Journal of the American Animal Hospital Association* 55:49–69.

Bone Loss

Bone loss can be localized in one particular area or generalized, where major sections of the crestal bone are involved. It can be either horizontal, where the marginal alveolar bone around adjacent teeth is decreased (Fig. 7.3), or vertical, with V-shaped alveolar bone defects on one or all roots (Fig. 7.4).

Furcation Exposure

Furcation exposure appears radiographically as an area of lucency due to loss of intraradicular bone (see "A" in Fig. 7.3).

Alveolar Dehiscence

Alveolar dehiscence occurs when there is a loss of the alveolar buccal bone. Radiographically, there is a break in the continuity of the lamina dura and loss of the

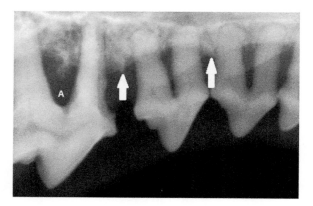

Figure 7.3 Radiograph of maxillary premolars. Note the horizontal bone loss (indicated by the arrows) that involves all the teeth shown.

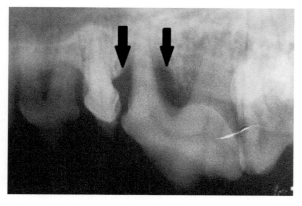

Figure 7.4 Radiograph of a maxillary fourth premolar (208). Note the vertical bone loss along the mesial buccal root (indicated by the arrows).

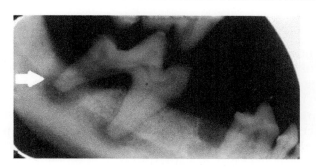

Figure 7.5   Radiograph of a mandibular first molar (409). Note the alveolar dehiscence that runs along the entire distal root (indicated by the arrow).

periodontal space. Alveolar bone loss can extend from the alveolar margin apically, involving the whole root[4] (Fig. 7.5).

Treatment and Therapies

Prevention versus Treatment

In veterinary dental literature, the use of more precise terminology is recommended for the description of the prevention and treatment of periodontal disease. It is essential for the dentistry staff to become familiar with these differences and implement them into their vocabulary, treatment protocols, and fees.

Remove the phrase "doing a dental" from the list. It does not specify the treatment or procedure being performed. The treatment plan details the procedures to be implemented. To use precise terminology, it is essential to understand the difference between a dental prophylaxis and a periodontal treatment.

On presentation, the oral cavity may have affected areas where only plaque is visible through to areas of gum recession and inflammation. Each mouth is to be treated tooth by tooth. A prophylaxis is a preventative treatment. A tooth with plaque and calculus and no gingival inflammation qualifies as a dental prophylaxis. If gingival inflammation, recession, periodontal pockets, furcation exposure, or mobility are present, a periodontal treatment needs to be performed (see web content: Video 7.1W Periodontal Hand Instrumentation).

The Goal of Periodontal Therapy

The goal of periodontal therapy is threefold. The first goal is the reduction of periodontal pockets or the elimination of soft tissue or bony lesions. The second goal is to slow or stop the progress of a periodontal lesion. The third goal is to return the tissues to a normal environment by removing all tooth deposits through professional cleanings and diligent home care.[5]

Periodontal pockets form due to the apical migration of plaque bacteria, causing destruction of soft and bony tissue. Over 50% attachment loss carries a poor prognosis. It is with professional treatments and rigorous home care that success can be seen (see web content: Presentation 7.1W Stages of periodontal disease).[2]

Flap Surgery

A flap is a section of tissue that has been cut and raised with one side still attached. Flaps are useful because they allow exposure of the root surface while maintaining the attached gingiva. They also enable the gingiva to be sutured in such a way that the pocket can be reduced.[6]

The objective of flap surgery is to allow adequate access and visibility to the diseased area. When making the flap, the base should be 1.5 times as wide as the coronal aspect to allow adequate blood flow. The flap needs to be sutured closed to prevent displacement, bleeding, hematoma formation, and infection.[6]

There are two types of flaps: full thickness and partial thickness. Full-thickness flaps are used to gain visibility for bony areas to perform procedures such as root planing and pocket elimination. A periosteal elevator is placed under the periosteum and rocked until it is peeled away from the bone. Partial-thickness flaps leave a layer of the periosteum. This procedure is used in areas where there are thin, bony plates, or in areas where there is dehiscence where bone must be protected or in areas where the bone loss is permanent (see web content: Presentation 7.2W Flap procedures).[6]

Regenerative Therapy

The goal of regenerative therapy is to keep the faster growing alveolar mucosa and gingival connective tissue out of the lesion to allow the growth of the periodontal ligament and bone. Osseopromotive products such as Consil (Nutramax, Baltimore, MD), which is a biosynthetic particulate glass material, act as a barrier and stimulate new bone growth.[2]

For regenerative therapy to be successful, all debris and granulation tissue must be removed to clean, healthy bone or tooth surface. Pre- and postoperative radiographs should be taken. Removal of any diseased marginal gingiva would also be beneficial. A full-thickness flap that includes attached gingiva may be necessary to close the lesion without any tension. These patients are reexamined at 10–14 days. A follow-up cleaning, exam, and radiographs is recommended 3–4 months later.[2]

Periodontal Splinting

When teeth are mobile, it decreases the chances of retention. If the plan is to try regenerative therapy, splinting the teeth may provide stability. This technique can also be used after a traumatic luxation or subluxation of a tooth. The teeth are cleaned and polished, and any debris or granulation tissue is removed. The osseopromotive product is placed in the defect and sutured closed. A band of dental acrylic is placed around the teeth in the area of the defect with stabile tooth on either side. The acrylic attaches one tooth to another for stabilization.[6]

The splinted area must be cleaned daily using rinses. Regular recheck must follow with a full oral exam with radiographs in 3–4 months.

Extraction or Exodontics

The role of dental radiology

Preoperative dental radiographs are necessary. Knowledge of abnormal anatomy and pathology will allow the steps of the extraction to be planned. Postoperative radiographs to assess the extraction should also be taken.

Types of extractions

There are two basic extraction techniques: (1) closed or nonsurgical, which involves simple luxation or elevation without the removal of alveolar bone; and (2) open or surgical, which involves raising a mucoperiosteal flap to reveal the alveolar bone. The flap is raised by making releasing incisions from the gingival margin to beyond the mucogingival line. Two-thirds of the root length of the alveolar bone is removed using a bur on a high-speed handpiece to expose the roots.[7] The exposed roots allow the doctor to have a purchase point to place a dental elevator and start elevating the tooth. The open technique can be used on all teeth and is recommended if the tooth is not mobile.

When working with multirooted teeth, it is best to section the tooth into single-rooted sections using a taper fissure bur on a high-speed handpiece. When sectioning a tooth, the gingival attachment to the tooth is incised to expose the furcation. The bur is inserted into the furcation and moved coronally, cutting into the crown (see web content: Presentation 7.3W Dental extractions).

When using a closed or open extraction technique, suturing the gingiva over the defect is recommended. Suturing reduces postoperative pain. The suture material should be absorbable on a reverse cutting needle. Common suture materials include 3-0 to 5-0 chromic gut and 3-0 to 5-0 poliglecaprone 25 (see web content: Video 7.2W Extraction instrumentation).

Oronasal Fistula

An oronasal fistula is a communication between the oral cavity and the nasal cavity. It can occur in different ways. With periodontal disease, the fistula occurs due to the continuous bone and attachment loss as the pathogenic bacteria moves down the root. Eventually, the bacteria erode the plate that separates the oral cavity from the nasal cavity.

Oronasal fistulas can occur with any tooth in the maxilla, but are most commonly associated with the canine tooth.

Symptoms of the presence of an oronasal fistula are chronic sneezing, sometimes with a purulent or bloody discharge. Dogs with a dolichocephalic head shape are most commonly affected, particularly dachshunds.[8]

Oronasal fistulas are diagnosed when the patient is under general anesthesia. A periodontal probe is the instrument of choice. The probe is inserted along the palatal aspect of the maxillary tooth. The periodontal probe will measure an abnormally deep pocket and bleeding may occur from the corresponding nostril. Another diagnostic indicator is to gently flush the pocket with saline; if the saline comes out of the corresponding nostril, there is communication (see web content: Presentation 7.4W Oronasal fistula).

Treatment of oronasal fistulas is extraction of the tooth or teeth in the area of the fistula. The extraction site must be thoroughly cleaned of debris and granulation tissue.

The gingiva is closed using a full-thickness mucoperiosteal flap so there is no tension. A long-lasting absorbable suture such as polyglactin 910 or poliglecaprone is used to close the tissue. Blood-tinged saliva and nasal discharge is common during the first 24–48 hours after surgery. Home care includes the use of antibiotics and pain medications.

Antibiotic Use in Periodontal Disease Treatment

Systemic antibiotics are not recommended for periodontal disease prevention. In a clean and healthy mouth, antibiotics could decrease beneficial, along with pathogenic, organisms.

Systemic antibiotics are recommended in eight patient scenarios:

- If the tissue around the teeth is severely infected, necessitating periodontal surgery or extraction
- If the infection has progressed to osteomyelitis despite oral surgery
- If severe ulceration and loss of mucosal integrity are present
- In patients who are immunosuppressed
- If the patient has had a splenectomy
- If the patient has a prosthetic device
- If the patient has severe systemic disease
- If the patient is having sterile surgeries on other parts of their body under the same anesthetic procedure.[9]

The most commonly used systemic antibiotics for the treatment of periodontal disease is clindamycin, amoxicillin/clavulanate, and doxycycline. Clindamycin and amoxicillin/clavulanate are the most effective against a large percentage of oral pathogens.

Locally applied antimicrobials or perioceutics do not subject the body to unnecessary antimicrobial exposure. The antimicrobial product used in perioceutics is either doxycycline or clindamycin in a biodegradable form that is placed in the affected periodontal pocket. It remains in the periodontal pocket for several weeks, slowly releasing therapeutic levels of the drug.[9,10]

Importance of Follow-Up Visits and Periodontal Maintenance

Oral and written home care instructions should be individualized to the patient (see Chapter 10). It is important to alert the client to possible side effects such as bleeding, coughing, nasal discharge, neurological signs, vomiting, diarrhea, anorexia, or signs of pain. Soft food should be fed either in the form of moistened hard food or canned food. Set up a recheck appointment for after the antibiotics have been taken.

The client should be called the day after surgery to inquire about the patient's condition, ability to give the medication, the patient's tolerance of the medication, and to answer any questions or concerns.

At the recheck appointment, the sutured areas are checked for signs of dehiscence or further infection. If the suture sites look healthy and healing is taking place, resume the patient's regular diet. The home care instructions are reviewed again and revised if necessary. Schedule more recheck appointments until the disease or wound is controlled – monthly to every 3 months.

Assess Your Patient and Your Client

The role of the veterinarian and the technician includes education, treatment, and support. Management of periodontal disease requires the building and nurturing of the relationship between the owner, animal, and the environment. The owner is the one who will be investing a high level of time and commitment. It is important that the owner feels that they are part of the treatment decisions that will best suit their pet based on their ability to carry out the treatment.[11]

In Conclusion

Prevention and treatment of periodontal disease is a common procedure in the veterinary practice. To maintain long-term oral hygiene or treat existing periodontal disease, input needs to come from the veterinary staff, the client, and the pet. The combination of practicing high-quality dentistry, updating your knowledge and treatment protocols, knowing when to refer, and solid client support should bring about a successful outcome for the patient.

With the presence of a veterinary technician specialty group in dentistry, the opportunities for technicians to gain further knowledge in this field are more available both at a local and at a national level. With periodontal disease being the most frequently clinically occurring condition in dogs and cats, it is imperative that the veterinary technician keep up with current information regarding pathogenesis, treatment options, and home care.

Part of what makes a veterinary technician an indispensable part of the medical staff is the ability to bridge the gap between the client and the veterinarian. Your level of professionalism is gauged by your knowledge and, more importantly, how well you can communicate your knowledge. Your medical knowledge of the procedures used in the prevention and treatment of periodontal disease involved is crucial.

Endodontic Disease

Sara Sharp, CVT, VTS (Dentistry)

Anatomy of the Pulp

The general definition of endodontics is the treatment of the pulp of the tooth. The pulp is made up of blood vessels, nerves, and connective tissue that help support the odontoblastic cells lining the pulp chamber of the tooth. The apex of each tooth has an opening called the apical delta. When a tooth becomes infected or traumatized, the animal is able to feel pain because of the nerves that run through the root apex. Infection is also able to spread from the inside of the tooth and from the outside of the tooth into the pulp.

Indications for Endodontic Therapy Due to Trauma

Indications for endodontic therapy due to trauma include the following:

- Discolored teeth – indicating possible necrosis of the pulp
- Fractured teeth with an exposed nonvital pulp
- Fractured teeth with an exposed vital pulp. These fractures are to be treated within a short period of time to avoid pulpal necrosis and/or to allow the pulp to continue to develop
- Fractured teeth with a "near" exposure causing sensitivity and increased chance of infection and further fracture

Preventative Endodontics

This treatment is provided for teeth that are at high risk of fracture. Patients that fall into this category are:

- Dogs that chew at cage doors, causing continual wear to the distal aspects of their canine teeth
- Police dogs that practice bite work on a hard sleeve, causing wear or possible fracture of the canine teeth. The canine teeth are the police dog's weapon and need to be protected
- Dogs that do agility or fly ball competition, where toys are constantly being carried, causing wear to the canine teeth

The Endodontic Exam

Animals with endodontic disease are painful. The dead and dying pulp of the tooth causes inflammation and infection, and thus pain receptors are stimulated, causing oral sensitivity and severe discomfort. Many pet owners do not perceive their animal's pain, however. Pets are able to hide their pain until they are no longer able to compensate, then the pain will manifest itself in symptoms.

Symptoms of oral pain include the following:

- Salivation
- Inappetance
- Lethargy
- Inability to eat or drink properly
- Odor
- Swelling/redness
- Draining lesions on the gingiva

- Reluctance to chew
- Inability to close the mouth properly
- Reluctance to play or be petted
- Changes in socialization
- Dropping of food while eating
- Vocalization with oral activity
- Ear and ocular pain
- Ocular discharge

A complete history needs to be taken, focusing on when the injury occurred or the abnormality was found. Treatment will involve the patient going under anesthesia. A full physical, oral exam, and presurgical blood work needs to be performed.

Once under anesthesia, each tooth must be assessed on an individual basis for disease, both visually and using dental radiographs. A full survey of dental radiographs should be performed on the patient during the assessment. This will help tell the veterinarian the health and stability of the affected tooth by looking at the pulp chamber of the tooth, the surrounding tissue, bone, and ligament. The pulp chamber size should be evaluated to see if the maturation process of the tooth has progressed at the same rate as the other teeth. As a tooth matures, the pulp chamber gets narrower. This is a good way to monitor if the maturation of the tooth was interrupted or stopped due to infection or damage. Radiographs will also show the presence of periapical lysis, degradation of the periodontal ligament, and integrity of the surrounding bone structure. All of these factors will help determine the severity of the endodontic disease and the likelihood of a successful endodontic treatment.

The Endodontic Treatment

The advantages of endodontic therapy include the following:

- Less invasive than extraction
- Recovery time is faster
- Integrity of jaw is stronger with the tooth in place
- Highly successful
- Very efficient procedure
- Cost is comparable to a surgical extraction

Types of Endodontic Therapy

- Vital pulp therapy
- Standard root canal therapy
- Surgical root canal therapy

Please note that before any of these procedures are performed, a local/regional nerve block is administered to the patient to help with pain control during the operation. A nerve block helps lessen the amount of gas anesthesia needed, and helps with postoperative pain control. See Chapter 4.

Patient and Treatment Considerations for Endodontic Therapy

If the animal does "mouth work" found in agility, field trials, and obedience, further damage to the tooth is possible. In this case, the crown may need to be partially amputated to take it out of occlusion, thus preventing further damage, or a metal crown needs to be placed after endodontic therapy. If the owner wants to keep the remaining crown intact, a crown or on-lay for this tooth could be placed to provide additional strength. A crown is not as strong as the original tooth; however, it will be stronger than not having protection to the crown. The considerations for crown therapy on fractured teeth include cost, further anesthetics to place the crown, and consideration of the oral activity of the pet. If the animal is unsupervised with oral activity, the crown may be lost, or the tooth could break further due to sheer force on the crown by inappropriate oral activity.

The environment, both external and internal, needs to be a consideration in vital pulp therapy. If the animal has severe periodontal disease, or if it comes from an external environment that is not clean, or has oral habits that are not sanitary, the owner may be encouraged to proceed with a standard root canal therapy as opposed to a vital pulp therapy due to the increase in bacterial exposure.

After determining all these factors, the veterinarian can help the client make an educated choice as to which procedure would be best for their animal.

Vital Pulp Therapy

Vital pulp therapy is a procedure used when the tooth has been freshly fractured and the pulp is still vital or living. The procedure is short. There are many factors that need to be taken into consideration when performing a vital pulp therapy. These include the following:

- The age of the animal
- The length of time the tooth has been fractured
- Which tooth has been fractured

The age of the animal must be considered because of the canal development. Apexogenesis may not be complete. Apexogenesis describes the completion of normal developmental root lengthening in young permanent vital teeth. This process may take up to 24 months.[12] If the animal is very young, less than 24 months of age, the pulp canal is still very wide and the apex of the root may not have closed. In young permanent teeth, the tooth walls are thin so the tooth is not very strong. An open apex will have to have an apexification performed first so that the apex will close and the tooth will continue to mature. Apexification is the process of stimulating the apex to close with hard tissue. This procedure is performed when a necrotic pulp is present in an incompletely developed young permanent tooth where normal tooth development is delayed by an infectious or noninfectious process.[12] It does not preclude a young animal from having more endodontic therapy in the future.

Apexification can be done by packing a thin layer of a lining material such as calcium hydroxide in the fracture site and placing a restoration filling on top. The calcium hydroxide will irritate and stimulate the pulp to close the apex of the tooth.

If necessary, the tooth can be reopened after this has occurred and standard root canal therapy performed.[13]

The length of time that the tooth has been fractured is also important. As long as the pulp is exposed to the outside environment, it is being exposed to bacteria that can infect the pulp. Vital pulp therapy should not be performed if the tooth has been fractured with pulp exposure for more than 48 hours. The owner must be warned that the vital pulp therapy can fail and that a standard or even surgical root canal may have to be performed at a later date. The tooth must be monitored for the lifetime of the animal.

The vital pulp therapy procedure is faster than standard root canal therapy because the pulp remains mostly intact. Sterility of the procedure is very important. Although the mouth is not sterile to begin with, we do not want to introduce further contamination so an aseptic environment should be maintained throughout the procedure.

The first step is to radiograph the tooth to determine the extent of damage to the tooth. If the crown is fractured and the root is intact, this tooth is a good candidate for vital pulp therapy. The integrity of the bone surrounding the tooth and the presence of any apical lesions should be checked. If there is a vertical crack or fracture in the tooth, further therapy may be required, including standard root canal therapy and a crown placement (Fig. 7.6).

Steps of the vital pulpotomy

1. After the radiograph has been taken, the mouth should be rinsed thoroughly to help cut the bacteria count and the affected tooth should be soaked for about 5 minutes with a chlorhexidine solution to help decrease the bacteria count.
2. A sterile bur and handpiece should be used to amputate the first 5 mm of the exposed pulp. The pulp should bleed profusely at this step. The area is then gently lavaged with cold sterile saline to help control hemorrhage.
3. A thin layer of a lining cement such as mineral trioxide aggregate (MTA) or calcium hydroxide is then placed. This irritates the pulp to form a bridge over the exposed pulp, thus giving a protective layer between it and the external environment (Fig. 7.7).

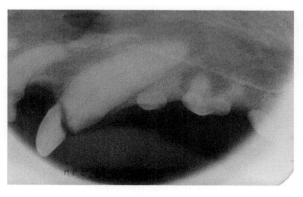

Figure 7.6　Fracture that happened 2 hours before the procedure. Bone and tooth structure both sound. Fractured tooth tip removed and vital pulpotomy performed.

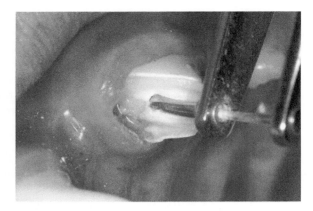

Figure 7.7   Mineral trioxide aggregate (MTA) placement into canal after amputating 5 mm of tooth root.

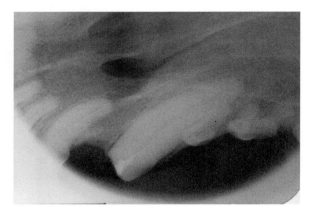

Figure 7.8   Final radiograph of completed vital pulpotomy.

4. An intermediate restorative layer such as a glass ionomer should then be placed over the layer of lining cement, providing a foundation between the cement liner that protects the pulp and the final restoration.
5. A final restoration is then placed over the cured glass ionomer and shaped and smoothed. After this is cured, a radiograph is then taken of the final restorations to make sure there are no air pockets present (Fig. 7.8).

The tooth should be radiographed after 6 months to check for further maturation of the pulp and also for signs of periapical disease. After that, the patient should be monitored yearly at each dental cleaning for continued signs of infection or death of the pulp.

Home care for the patient should include a few days' course of nonsteroidal anti-inflammatory drugs (NSAIDs) to help cut down on inflammation and pain. The client should also monitor the tooth weekly for signs of discoloration, further damage, fistula formation on the gingiva above the affected tooth, and signs of pain. If any of these signs occur, the patient should be anesthetized and radiographed to see if the vital pulp therapy may be failing.

Standard Root Canal Therapy

Standard root canal therapy involves removal of all of the pulp and nerve, disinfecting the canal, and filling the canal and filling and capping it. This procedure will make the tooth nonvital but in doing so will remove pain and allow the animal to keep the tooth, maintaining normal dental occlusion.

A standard root canal should be performed if a tooth has been fractured for more than 48 hours or if it has been determined that the pulp may already be contaminated and is nonvital.

Steps of the standard root canal therapy

1. The patient should be anesthetized and radiographs taken to determine the amount of damage sustained and the apex evaluated for signs of periapical disease and/or root fracture or disease (Fig. 7.9).
2. If the radiograph shows that the animal is a good candidate for a standard root canal therapy, the affected tooth should be disinfected and asepsis should be maintained.
3. A direct access site into the pulp through the tooth surface needs to be established. This will help with accessibility to the natural curve of the tooth root and prevent strain and stress on the files that will be used, thus preventing separation of the file or breakage of the file within the tooth (Fig. 7.10).
4. There are many types of files that can be used to help remove the nerve and pulp from the tooth. The files each have a different function. They also come in many lengths to fit many canal sizes. The Hedstrom file is used in a push/pull motion. The K-file is used in a twisting motion; the barbed broach can be used to "snag" the pulp.
5. An ethylenediaminetetraacetic acid (EDTA) preparation is a chelating compound that can be used to help lubricate the files and softens the dentin.
6. A radiograph should be taken when the file reaches the apex of the root to be sure that it is all the way down to the apex and to check that it has not gone past the apex of the tooth (see web content: Fig. 7.11W).

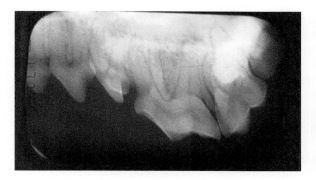

Figure 7.9   Radiograph of tooth prior to root canal treatment to check for integrity of bone and apex. Note the apical abscess present on the distal root of 208.

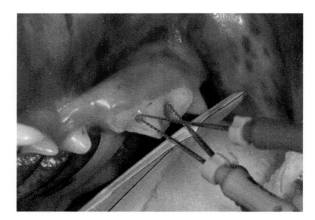

Figure 7.10 All files are placed in the canals for the master file radiograph checking for depth of the files.

7. A 6% solution of sodium hypochlorite (household bleach) should be infused into the canal and left to stand for approximately 5 minutes. This will help with canal disinfection. It will infuse into all lateral canals and help to soften any additional debris left behind.

8. The sodium hypochlorite solution is then flushed out with sterile saline and the debrided canal is dried with paper points. Paper points are rolled pieces of paper that are conical shaped and sized to fit canal sizes. The canal should be thoroughly dried and no sign of blood or pulp should be noted. If debris is still seen, the filing process should be resumed until the canal is clean and flushed.

9. A sealant material is placed into the clean canal. This mixture will help with sealing the lateral canals and provides an improved apical seal. Gutta percha is a rubber-based material that is used to help fill the canal after cleaning and sealing.

10. Gutta percha comes in many forms – solid points or liquid. A three-dimensional fill is desired. The goal of the placement of the gutta percha is to provide a nonirritating, inert fluid tight seal in the pulp chamber. Radiographs are taken during the filling procedure to determine that the material is reaching the apex of the canal and the gutta percha is providing a tight seal. If there are voids in the gutta percha, or if it extends past the end of the apex, the process will need to be started over until a good obturation or filling of the canal is complete (see web content: Fig. 7.12W).

11. A glass ionomer is then placed over the gutta percha, forming an intermediate layer between the filling material and the final restoration.

12. A final restoration is placed on top of the glass ionomer and a radiograph taken of the final work. Again, voids or air bubbles should be noted and restorations may need to be replaced if any are present (see web content: Figs. 7.13W and 7.14W).

Aftercare for the root canal patient may consist of NSAIDs for a few days to help relieve any inflammation and also for any temporomandibular joint (TMJ) pain that they may incur. Antibiotics should not be needed unless they are indicated for an apical abscess. The final filling should be checked after a month and the owners should be instructed to also monitor the filling and the gingiva above the tooth for any fistula formation, swelling, or pain. A radiograph should be taken after 6 months to check for apical abscess. Yearly radiographs should be taken to monitor the tooth throughout the life of the patient.

Surgical Root Canal Therapy

A surgical root canal can be performed along with a standard root canal therapy when there is disease of the apex of the root. If, upon radiographing the tooth, the apex of the tooth is open, or if there is an apical disease or destruction is present, then a standard root canal therapy and a surgical root canal therapy could be performed (see web content: Fig. 7.15W).

1. Following the conclusion of the standard root canal therapy, a "window" is opened in the gingiva and bone overlying the apex of the tooth where the abscess is located.
2. A gingival flap is made and reflected back, exposing the bone. The bone is then drilled away until the apex of the tooth is exposed.
3. The area is then curetted and all the granulation and diseased tissue is debrided. The area is then flushed thoroughly and dried. The apex of the tooth root is amputated (about 2–3 mm) and a cement material is placed in the apex of the root, thus sealing it off from top and bottom. Once the cement is in place, the gingiva is then sutured back over the "window" and a radiograph is taken of the finished procedure.

The animal will need to be monitored closely for signs of failure of the procedure. Owners should watch for pain, swelling, and fistula formation over the apex of the tooth root on the gingiva. If this occurs, the tooth will probably need to be extracted. Failure rate of a surgical root canal therapy is slightly higher than that of a standard root canal due to the presence of infection at the root tip. We are unable to tell if all infection has been removed during the procedure. Aftercare of the patient should involve not only NSAIDs for swelling and pain but also a course of an appropriate antibiotic. A radiograph should be taken at 6 months and then yearly after to monitor the stability of the tooth.

In Conclusion

Have information available and give owners all options when making a decision. There is information available on the website of the AVDC (www.avdc.org), the Foundation for Veterinary Dentistry (https://www.veterinarydentistry.org/), and the Academy of Veterinary Dental Technicians (www.avdt.us). Be sure to supply owners with appropriate handouts and websites for them to research on their own also.

When recommending endodontic procedures, it is important to educate the owner of all options that are available. Remember, it is best to try and save teeth whenever possible. Extraction should be the last option.

Malocclusion

Patricia A. March, RVT, VTS (Dentistry)

Normal Occlusion

A normal or "ideal" occlusion is described as the perfect alignment or interdigitation between the upper and the lower teeth, when the mouth is closed[14] (Figs. 7.16 and 7.17). This occurs because the maxilla is longer and wider than the mandible. The maxillary incisors will be in a rostral position to the mandibular incisor teeth. The mandibular incisors rest on the enamel or "cingulum." The mandibular canines will be positioned between the maxillary third incisors and the maxillary canines, called the "dental interlock."[15] The premolar teeth will occlude in a specific pattern, not overlapping, but interdigitating. This effect has been termed a "pinking shear effect."[16] There will also be a very close alignment of the developmental grooves of the maxillary fourth premolars and the mandibular first molars.

Several factors may affect jaw occlusion, such as nutrition, environment, trauma, and genetics. Genetics should be considered when taking into account the normal size and shape of the head of certain breeds of dogs and cats.

- Brachycephalic breeds, such as bulldogs, boxers, pugs, and Burmese and Persian cats, have a shortened maxilla with crowded and rotated teeth. This abnormality results from chondrodystrophy of the chondrocranium rather than an overgrowth of the mandible.[17]

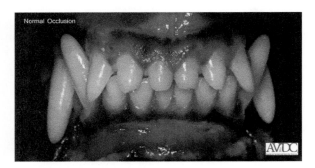

Figure 7.16 Normal occlusion (Copyright AVDC, used with permission).

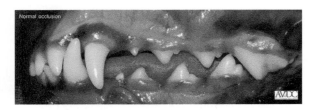

Figure 7.17 Normal occlusion (Copyright AVDC, used with permission).

- Mesocephalic or mesatocephalic breeds, such as German shepherds and Labrador retrievers, have a well-proportioned head where the maxilla is longer and wider than the mandible. The teeth are evenly spaced and in a normal occlusion, called a "scissor bite."[18]
- Dolichocephalic breeds, such as greyhounds and Shetland sheepdogs, have an elongated muzzle with increased interdental spaces or diastema between the premolars.

A malocclusion is defined as any deviation of the normal occlusion.[14] This condition may occur due to congenital or hereditary factors causing irregularity of the jaw bones, or teeth erupting in an abnormal position. These abnormalities will typically appear after eruption of the deciduous teeth, and may be noticed during the eruption of the permanent dentition. A malocclusion involving the deciduous teeth will likely result in permanent malocclusion if action is not taken. As a technician, you should become familiar with the eruption times and spatial arrangements of the teeth. This will allow you to become more adept at noticing signs of possible malocclusions and bringing them to the veterinarian's attention. The eruption process may also be compromised, delaying or impeding deciduous and/or permanent teeth eruption. Due to the crowding or misalignment of the teeth causing accumulation of plaque and debris, animals with malocclusion are predisposed to periodontal disease. These malpositioned teeth may cause soft tissue defects to the palate, the floor of the mouth, and oronasal fistula formation or gingival trauma. Fracture or excessive wearing or attrition due to improper tooth contact may also occur.

Types and Treatments of Malocclusions

Malocclusions are divided into symmetrical and asymmetrical skeletal malocclusions.

Symmetrical Skeletal Malocclusions

Class I malocclusion (MAL/1) or neutrocclusion

Class I malocclusion (MAL/1) or neutrocclusion is defined as a normal relationship between the maxilla and the mandible, with one or more teeth out of alignment.[14] Examples include the following:

- **Base-narrow canine or "lingually displaced mandibular canine":** This is a condition where the crown tip or cusp of the mandibular canine tooth or teeth come in contact with the palate in a lingual position. This type of malocclusion may be due to persistent deciduous mandibular canine teeth.
- **Base-wide mandibular canine:** This occurs when the mandibular canine tooth or teeth flare out in a lateral position. This is often associated with lancing maxillary canines and may lead to the inability to lift certain portions of the lips and protruding tips of the canine teeth. Prolonged exposure of the teeth can cause drying or desiccation of the crown tips, which may result in tooth discoloration.

■ **Lance canine:** This is a mesioversion or retroversion of the maxillary canine tooth, is often due to a lack of or a decreased diastema between the third incisors and the maxillary canines. This condition is very common in Shetland sheepdogs.

■ **Rostral crossbite:** This occurs when the maxillary incisors are displaced palatally and/or the mandibular incisor teeth are displaced labially.

■ **Caudal crossbite:** This is diagnosed when there is an improper, reversed relationship between the maxillary fourth premolar and the mandibular first molar. This condition is common in sight hounds, collies, Irish terriers, and petit basset griffon vendeens (see web content: Fig. 7.18W).

Class II malocclusion (MAL/2) or mandibular distocclusion

Class II malocclusion is defined as a mandible that is shorter than average.[14] This common malocclusion has often been referred to by the terms "overjet," "overbite," "undershot," or "mandibular brachygnathism." Teeth may be improperly aligned or malpositioned (see web content: Figs. 7.19W and 7.20W).

Class III malocclusion (MAL/3) or mandibular mesiocclusion

Class III malocclusion is defined as a mandible that is longer than normal.[14] This type of malocclusion has often been referred to as "reverse scissor bite," "prognathism," or "underbite." Brachycephalic dogs and cats are frequently placed in this category, although there is normally an abnormal relationship between the maxilla and mandible. When the mouth is in a closed position, the maxillary and mandibular incisors meet in a level or even bite. When the maxillary incisors align on the lingual aspects of the mandibular incisors when the mouth is closed, this is often referred to as a "reverse scissor bite" (see web content: Figs. 7.21W and 7.22W).[15]

Asymmetrical Skeletal Malocclusions

Asymmetrical skeletal malocclusions occur when there is a malocclusion or malpositioning of individual teeth[14] (Table 7.3).

Asymmetrical skeletal malocclusions are further subdivided into the direction of movement, such as rostrocaudal, side-to-side, or dorsoventral:

■ Maxillary-mandibular asymmetry in a rostrocaudal direction is seen when there is a mandibular mesiocclusion or distocclusion present only on one side of the face.[14]

■ Maxillary-mandibular asymmetry in a side-to-side direction is seen where there is a loss of normal midline alignment between the maxilla and the mandible. The term "wry bite," which previously was categorized as a Class IV malocclusion, is no longer recommended due to its nonspecificity.[14]

■ Maxillary-mandibular asymmetry in a dorsoventral direction is seen when there is an abnormal vertical spacing between the left and right sides of the mouth when it is in a closed position. It is also called and "open bite" (OB).

Table 7.3   Dental malocclusions

- Distoversion (DV) is the correct term for a tooth that is abnormally angled in a caudal direction
- Mesioversion (MV) is used to describe a tooth that is abnormally angled toward the midline
- Linguoversion (LV) should be used to identify a mandibular tooth that is abnormally angled toward the tongue
- Labioversion (LABV) is the proper term for an incisor or canine tooth that is abnormally angled toward the lips
- Buccoversion (BV) is a more precise term used to describe a premolar or molar tooth that is abnormally angled toward the cheek
- Crossbite (XB) is a term used when there is an abnormal positioning between the maxillary tooth or teeth and the mandibular tooth or teeth. This abnormal position may be in a buccal or a labial direction
- Rostral crossbite (RXB) is when one or more mandibular incisors are labial to the maxillary incisors when the mouth is in the closed position. This was previously called "anterior crossbite"
- Caudal crossbite (CXB) is when one or more mandibular cheek teeth are buccal to the maxillary cheek teeth when the mouth is in a closed position. This used to be called "posterior crossbite"

Position Statements

The American Veterinary Medical Association (AVMA) states that the correction of a conformational defect in a dog or cat is unethical, except when that abnormality affects the health and/or welfare of the animal.

The AVDC states that the goal of an orthodontic procedure is to provide pets with a healthy and functional occlusion. The AVDC supports the AVMA policy regarding cosmetic procedures that enhance the appearance of show or breeding animals.

The American Kennel Club (AKC) declares it is illegal to show a dog whose conformation has been altered in any way. The AKC (www.akc.org) has standards relating to dental corrections, stating that "a dog is considered changed in appearance by artificial means if it has been subjected to any type of procedure that has the effect of obscuring, disguising, or eliminating any congenital or hereditary abnormality or any undesirable characteristic or that does anything to improve a dog's natural appearance, temperament, bite, or gait. ... These procedures include: restorative dental procedures, the use of bands or braces on teeth, or any alteration of the dental arcade."[19]

Treatment of Malocclusions

The principle of orthodontic movement involves the use of force. Force is applied to the crowns of the teeth, which exerts on the roots, which press against the alveolar bone. The goal of treatment of malocclusions is to restore a functional bite.

The bone is reabsorbed at the side where there is pressure and new bone is laid down on the tension side. This will lead to the tooth gradually moving.[20] Light, continuous forces result in more rapid (physiological) tooth movement and less patient discomfort, whereas heavy, continuous forces will result in pathological movement or damage to both the tooth and the periodontal tissues.[21]

The goal of treatment is to restore a functional bite. This is accomplished by diagnosing the malocclusion early and preventing the various problems that may occur due to the abnormal bite.

Diagnosis is accomplished via a thorough oral examination and intraoral radiographs. If an animal's bite is considered functional and nontraumatic, treatment may not be necessary. The decision to provide orthodontic treatment is usually based on prevention of improper contact trauma, wear, or injury to hard or soft tissue.[16] Other options to orthodontic movement are vital pulp therapy and crown amputation, standard root canal therapy, or extraction of the affected tooth or teeth. Orthodontic treatment may take several months. Complications may include damage to permanent tooth buds, root resorption, root ankylosis, and overcorrection and malpositioning of affected teeth.

Common equipment used in orthodontics includes orthodontic wire, buttons, bands, elastomeric chains, wire twisters, acrylic composite material, acid-etch, enamel bonding material, brushes, light-cure gun, and nonfluoridated polish.

There are two main types of orthodontic treatment – interceptive and corrective.

Interceptive Orthodontics

Interceptive orthodontics is the process of removing improperly aligned deciduous teeth in the hopes of preventing further problems as the patient ages and the jaws continue to grow. If an animal has deciduous teeth in malocclusion, the affected teeth are extracted between 4 and 6 weeks prior to the expected permanent tooth eruption.

Corrective Orthodontics

When deciding to administer corrective orthodontics in a pure-breed animal, there are certain ethical considerations. The AVDC has issued a position statement:

> In cases of rostral crossbite, odontoplasty performed on permanent teeth in an attempt to alleviate crowding or a labial maxillary arch bar, with button brackets and elastic ligatures or chains may be used to move the maxillary incisors forward. Other options would be the use of a lingual maxillary arch bar with finger spring, a mandibular and maxillary incline plane, a maxillary expansion screw appliance or mandibular brackets and elastic chains. Extraction of the affected teeth is also an option.

If there is mild caudal crossbite, gingivoplasty or partial gingivectomy in the diastema may prevent contact trauma, pain, discomfort, and possible oronasal fistula formation. If the malocclusion is significant, then an orthodontic appliance, such as an inclined plane, with expansion springs and screws, is recommended. This procedure will help guide a more significant deviation, "tipping" the tooth to a functional location or normal occlusion is achieved.[16] This type of correction may be very prolonged and costly.

Base-wide canine teeth

Base-wide canine teeth may not require any intervention. If treatment is warranted, buttons or brackets with elastic ligatures are recommended to pull the teeth into a more lingual position.

Lance teeth

Lance teeth may be treated by extraction or orthodontic treatment. The orthodontic procedure begins with the scaling and polishing of the teeth with flour pumice. The crowns are then dried and prepped with acid-etch. Next, the buttons/brackets are applied with cement toward the tip of the canine that needs to be moved, called the target tooth and on the anchor teeth, typically the maxillary premolar and molars. A power chain or elastic ligature is placed between the target and the anchor teeth. These cases have to be monitored carefully to avoid the potential movement of the anchor teeth, usually weekly checkups until movement is complete. This process may take several months, especially in animals older than 1 year (see web content: Figs. 7.23W and 7.24W).

Base-narrow canine teeth

Base-narrow canine teeth or lingually displaced mandibular canine teeth may be treated by extraction of the affected tooth or teeth, vital pulpotomy and crown reduction, gingival wedge resection, or orthodontic treatment, such as a bite plate or a custom cast appliance. Passive ball therapy, allowing a young dog to chew on a properly sized rubber ball for several hours daily, has been used in mild cases with mixed results (see web content: Figs. 7.25W–7.30W).[22]

Types of Appliances

There are several different versions of orthodontic appliances: intraoral appliances, direct bonding, and fixed appliances, such as acrylic splints, expansion splints and bands, hooks, or buttons.

Direct acrylic appliance

A direct acrylic appliance, or inclined plane, is constructed in the oral cavity. This type of device may cause soft tissue irritation. The first part of the procedure is to ensure the crowns are clean, scaled, and polished with nonfluoridated polish or pumice. Acid-etch is applied to anchor teeth.

Dental acrylic is applied to both sides of the teeth, allowing it to flow in the diastema. While the acrylic material is still soft, it should be shaped accordingly to allow for proper alignment. When it is hardened, the composite should be trimmed and shaped so that no rough edges exist. The inclined plane may also be made by wrapping a figure-of-eight wire around the canine teeth, then covering the wire with acrylic and/or composite material. This procedure will move the canine teeth into a more normal alignment. The inclined plane may be left in place for several months and requires diligent home care by the owner (see web content: Figs. 7.31W and 7.32W).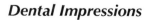

Dental Impressions

Dental impressions will be taken if an appliance needs to be fabricated by a laboratory. The procedure involves using plastic or metal impression trays, lined with alginate impression material. The filled trays are pressed over the dental arcade, held in place for up to 5 minutes, removed, rinsed, and allowed to harden. After the impressions are set, dental stone material is poured into the impression and left to harden. After a minimum of 45 minutes, the stone model is removed from the mold.

A bite registry is needed to determine the relationship of the maxilla and mandible. The registry is taken with a slab of softened bite wax, pressed between the maxilla and mandibular teeth. This should be performed prior to intubation or just after extubation.

In Conclusion

Unfortunately, orthodontic movement may be a long drawn out process whose outcome cannot be guaranteed. The client needs to be informed that there may be a need for frequent recheck examinations and sometimes intensive home care, such as cleansing an appliance daily, or adjusting the appliance weekly. Treatments may sometimes displace or damage normal teeth. The pet owner needs to be aware of which teeth are affected, the expected outcome, and how to care for the appliances. This is where the technician is an essential part of the dental team. There are several types of malocclusions and just as many treatment options. It is the responsibility of the veterinary technician to be familiar with both.

Jaw Fracture Management

Patricia A. March, RVT, VTS (Dentistry)

A fracture is defined as a break, split, or discontinuity in a bony structure. Fractures are further classified as closed, comminuted, complicated, greenstick, impacted, or open. A closed fracture is one in which the bone is broken, but the soft tissue is intact. With a comminuted fracture, there will be several pieces of broken bone. A complicated fracture will involve significant injury to organs, blood vessels, or nerves. A greenstick fracture will involve only one side of the bone; it is not a thorough break. When two fragments of a bone are jammed together, it is considered an impacted fracture. With an open fracture, there will be one or more pieces of bone breaking through the skin.

Types of Jaw Fractures and Their Treatment

The dog or cat skull consists of 35 bones and over 40 major foramina. The mandibles are subjected to opposing forces by the action of the jaw muscles, opening and closing the mouth,[23] which makes the mandibles the most common site of jaw fractures. Fractures occur at the mandibular symphysis, the coronoid or condylar processes, at the junction of the ramus and the body, and along the body of the mandible.[24]

A symphyseal separation is commonly seen in cats with a history of trauma. This is not a true fracture, but a type of joint instability.[24] In most cats, the mandibular

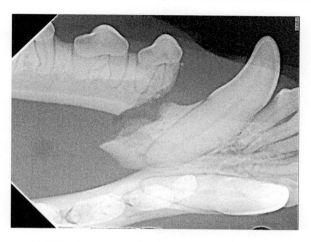

Figure 7.33 A 12-year-old Chihuahua presented for mandibular fracture. This is an example of a pathologic fracture due to severe periodontal disease (Reproduced with permission of Dr. Ira Luskin, Animal Dental Centers).

symphysis is a cartilaginous joint which never completely fuses, allowing for manual manipulation due to a laxity of the joint.

Fractures of the mandible may be further classified by involvement with a tooth: whether they encompass the bone and the tooth root, the bone and the apex of the tooth, or the bone with tooth root exposure.[25]

Jaw fractures may be traumatic or pathological in origin. The most common cause of jaw fracture is trauma. Pathological jaw fractures involve weakening of the jaws predisposing a particular animal to fracture due to severe periodontal disease or malignant oral tumors[24,26] (Fig. 7.33). Other causes of weakening of the jaw bones include metabolic disorders such as renal secondary hyperparathyroidism, nutritional secondary hyperparathyroidism, fungal infections, and osteogenesis imperfecta.[27]

Diagnosis of Jaw Fractures

Diagnosis of jaw fractures is made through a careful oral examination and history. Common symptoms are pain, swelling, bruising, epistaxis, bloody saliva, inability to eat or drink water, tilting of the head, and holding the mouth open or in an abnormal position[23,25] (Fig. 7.34). Intraoral radiographs are more desirable than head radiographs. If multiple maxillary and/or palatal fractures are suspected, a computed tomography (CT) scan may be advised to highlight both hard and soft tissue trauma.[24,28]

Jaw Fracture Management

In order to properly manage jaw fractures, several items should be considered. Alignment of the jaws to allow for the teeth to return to normal occlusion is necessary.[25] Any diseased or damaged teeth in the fracture site should be removed prior to

(a)　　　　　　　　　　　　　　　　　(b)

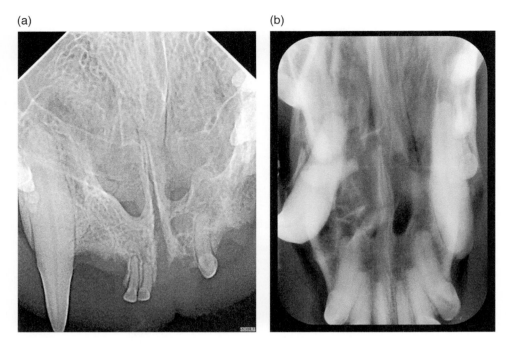

Figure 7.34 (a) An 8-year old domestic shorthair presented for maxillary fracture. The fractures were caused when the patient was hit by a car (Reproduced with permission of Dr. Ira Luskin, Animal Dental Centers). (b) A 6-year-old retriever presented for maxillary fracture. The fractures were caused when the patient was hit by a car (Reproduced with permission of Dr. Ira Luskin, Animal Dental Centers).

jaw fracture repair. If the tooth root is involved, consider root canal therapy to prevent a nonunion due to infection. Debride, lavage, and close soft tissue defects over the fracture site prior to stabilization. Extensive home care, such as feeding tube care, might be needed.[24,27,28]

Jaw Fracture Repair

Common methods of jaw fracture fixation include maxillomandibular fixation, circumferential wiring, interdental wiring, intraoral splinting, transosseous wiring, external skeletal fixation, bone plating, and partial mandibulectomy or maxillectomy.[28]

A tape muzzle may be utilized to treat minor unilateral mandibular fractures in young animals. This technique will help keep the jaws stabilized and the teeth in normal occlusion, or may be used as a temporary support until surgical repair can be performed. White cotton tape is fashioned in a band encircling the muzzle, leaving a 5–10 mm space to allow the tongue to protrude, with connecting bands on the sides of the face and extending behind the head. A piece of tape may also be applied between the eyes over the forehead. A regular fabric muzzle could also be used. This can be combined with acrylic crown extensions to hold the jaws in proper occlusion and prevent the jaws from shifting. The key is to allow the animal room to move the tongue, but not to open the jaws. With the muzzle on, they can lap up water and a liquefied diet. The muzzle will need to be changed often, as moist dermatitis may develop under the tape (see web content: Fig. 7.35W and Presentation 7.5W Tape muzzle).[23–25]

Interarcade acrylic bonding, or maxillomandibular fixation, is performed by applying acrylic between the maxillary and the mandibular canine teeth to stabilize jaw fractures. Interdental wires or elastics and buttons can also be used. When the canines are bonded together, there should be enough to space to allow the lapping of food and water, but not allowing for opening the jaws. In dogs, the distance between the maxillary and mandibular incisors should be between 1.0 and 2.0 cm, with the distance being 0.5–1.0 cm in cats. An esophagostomy feeding tube is often placed until the animal learns how to eat and drink on its own (see web content: Figs. 7.36W–7.38W).[24]

In cases of severe trauma, infection, necrosis, or pathological fractures due to periodontal disease, surgical removal such as partial mandibulectomy or maxillectomy may be warranted.[27,28] Bone grafting may be necessary if the removal will leave too large a bony defect.

Transosseous or interfragmentary wiring is performed only if the tooth roots will not be compromised by the wire placement or in areas of the mandible that do not have teeth.[24,27]

Interdental wiring is a technique used to stabilize adjacent teeth or several teeth in one quadrant. The basic technique involves looping the wire between and around the teeth, and may be extended to include all the teeth in one quadrant to improve stability.[23,24]

Fractures of the maxilla can range in severity and treatment options. Because of the thin maxillary bone and the close proximity of the nasal cavity, bone plates and intramedullary pins are contraindicated. For some fractures, interdental wiring and an acrylic splint may be required to stabilize areas of the maxilla and/or palate (see web content: Figs. 7.39W and 7.40W).[26,27]

Circumferential mandibular wiring is commonly used to repair symphyseal separation in cats and fractures located near the mandibular symphysis. The technique involves placement of wire around both mandibles, caudal to the canine teeth, and tightening it under the chin. The wire is left in place for up to 4 weeks and then removed. If the jaw is still unstable, a figure-of-eight pattern can be placed surrounding the canine teeth. An acrylic splint may be placed over the wire to ensure stabilization and to cover the sharp ends of the wire. The splint is typically left in place up to 8 weeks (see web content: Figs. 7.41W–7.43W).[24–28]

Intraoral splinting is accomplished when acrylic is applied to teeth along either side of the fracture to provide a rigid, interfragmentary fixation. The acrylic material is applied to the buccal surface of the maxilla for stabilization and to prevent palatal trauma from the splint material, as well as to achieve normal occlusion. If the fracture is located on the mandible, the acrylic should be applied to the lingual aspect of the mandibular teeth. The teeth are scaled and polished prior to placement of the acrylic. Next, the crowns are acid-etched and dried, and the acrylic is applied in layers or "spot bonding" which may improve the adhesion of the acrylic. You should check the occlusion frequently. Wire can be placed in a circumferential pattern, incorporating the wire within the acrylic to provide more stabilization near the fracture site. The acrylic will need to be shaped with burs to ensure a smooth, even surface. The splint is typically removed within 4–8 weeks, depending on how severe the fracture was and the age and health status of the patient. Removal of the splint is typically accomplished with the use of a high-speed bur and wire-cutting forceps. Extraction forceps may also be used to remove large chunks of the acrylic splint. The crowns of the teeth might require touch-up scaling and polishing.[23–29]

Bone plates, screws, and intermedullary pins are not commonly used due to the location of the mandibular tooth roots. The incorrect use of these types of fixtures could lead to damage of the inferior alveolar blood vessels, nerves, as well as the vitality of the teeth.[23–25] If a plate is deemed necessary, a maxillofacial miniplate is recommended, using screws of 1.5 or 2.0 mm diameter. A tape muzzle will often be recommended for several weeks.

External skeletal fixation may be used in cases of comminuted fractures or where there are large bony defects. This may be accomplished with the use of Kirschner wires, small Steinmann pins, and/or an acrylic splint. In these cases, the intermedullary pins should be placed between the tooth and/or the roots to avoid future problems.[23–25,27–29]

Patients with extensive facial trauma should be checked for fractures in the TMJ area, ideally with a CT scan. Fractures of the condylar or coronoid process may be treated conservatively, carefully watching for the possibility of the development of joint ankylosis. This may require future surgery.[24]

Home Care

Home care instructions are essential in jaw fracture management. There are several options for pain control in dogs. Cats may benefit from injectable NSAIDs, gabapentin, tramadol, oral buprenorphine, and fentanyl patches. Antibiotics are usually dispensed if they can be given with a minimum of oral manipulation, such as through a feeding tube. The oral cavity will need to be rinsed daily with an antibacterial solution to prevent gingivitis or oral ulcers. Canned food or softened dry food needs to be given; no toys or hard treats.[24]

Rechecks are usually done weekly, then every 2 weeks, and again at 4–8 weeks, requiring anesthesia and radiographs, plus splint removal.[24]

Possible complications include malocclusions from the jaws healing in an abnormal position, osteomyelitis, damage to teeth, ankylosis of the TMJ from the muzzle or maxillary mandibular fixation for extended periods, and possible feeding tube complications such as infection or expelling the feeding tube.[24,25]

Oral Tumors

Patricia A. March, RVT, VTS (Dentistry)

A tumor is defined as an abnormal mass of tissue that is not inflammatory, arises without obvious cause from cells of preexistent tissue, and possesses no physiological function. It may also be called a mass or neoplasm.[30]

In dogs and cats, the fourth most common site for neoplasia is the oral cavity.[31–33] Oral tumors can originate from numerous sites within the oral cavity, such as the mucosa, the tongue, the periodontium, the maxilla, the mandible, and the lips.[33] Oral tumors typically spread by direct extension or invasion of the adjacent bone and cartilaginous tissues. Metastasis occurs within the regional lymph nodes and lungs.[32]

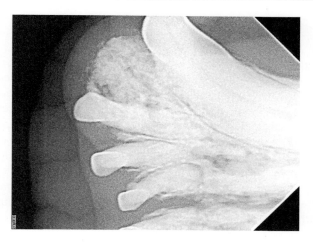

Figure 7.44 An 8-year-old pitbull presented with an oral mass. Diagnosis: peripheral odontogenic fibroma (Reproduced with permission of Dr. Ira Luskin, Animal Dental Centers).

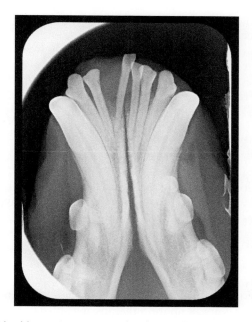

Figure 7.45 A 3-year-old golden retriever presented with an oral mass causing the mandibular incisors to move out of position. Diagnosis: acanthomatous ameloblastoma (Reproduced with permission of Dr. Ira Luskin, Animal Dental Centers).

Common symptoms of oral masses are visible swellings, oral bleeding, dysphasia, halitosis, weight loss, hypersalivation, nasal discharge, and enlargement of the regional lymph nodes. Upon examination, the oral mass may be visualized, along with loose teeth and facial deformities (Figs. 7.44 and 7.45).[31,33]

When attempting to identify an oral mass, be sure to take into account the normal anatomical structures; specifically, the lingual molar glands in cats, located medially to the first mandibular molars, the incisive papilla found on the rostral midline of the hard palate, and the normal papillae of the tongue (see web content: Fig. 7.46W).

Benign Oral Tumors and Treatments

The diagnostic approach begins with a complete physical examination and a limited, conscious intraoral examination. Other tests that should be included are complete blood count (CBC), chemistry panel, chest radiographs, electrocardiogram/echocardiogram, and aspirates of the palpable lymph nodes.[32,33] General anesthesia will be required for ultrasound-guided aspirates of the retropharyngeal lymph nodes, CT or magnetic resonance imaging (MRI), incisional biopsy, and intraoral radiographs.[31]

Benign oral tumors are unlikely to metastasize and tend to be less locally invasive. However, there are benign oral tumors that are locally aggressive, such as the acanthomatous ameloblastoma and papillary squamous cell carcinoma, which affect young dogs. There are several types of benign oral tumors: peripheral odontogenic fibromas, odontomas, gingival hyperplasia, and papillomas.[31,33]

Peripheral Odontogenic Fibromas

Peripheral odontogenic fibromas, previously referred to as epulides, are of a fibromatous or ossifying type.[33] These benign tumors are typically slow growing, may be smooth or pedunculated in appearance, and are usually found arising from the gingival tissues in middle-aged to older dogs.[31] The ossifying type will have an osteoid matrix. Intraoral radiographs are necessary to ensure the health of the teeth and the surrounding bone. Treatment is typically excision, but recurrence is common (see web content: Fig. 7.47W).[33]

Acanthomatous Ameloblastoma

Acanthomatous ameloblastomas are tumors that originate from the odontogenic tissues and while they do not metastasize, they are locally invasive and aggressive.[31,33] This type of tumor, seen as a smooth, firm, nonulcerated mass, is commonly found on the rostral mandible and occasionally on the maxilla, in middle-aged to older dogs.[31] Oral radiographs will show bone lysis, seen as a radiolucent area.[31] A rare, malignant form may occur, whose symptomology is similar to the benign form. Histopathology is necessary to ensure the diagnosis and treatment plan.[33] The recommended treatment is a large excisional biopsy, with 1–2 cm margins and removal of any teeth in direct contact with the tumor. Radiation therapy may also be an option.[31] New information suggests radiation therapy can lead to malignant transformation (see web content: Figs. 7.48W and 7.49W).

Odontomas

Odontomas are benign tumors that arise from the dental follicle, early in the stages of development of the teeth.[31] They may be compound, with multicellular differentiation and having toothlike structures, commonly known as "denticles" present within the mass or complex, in which the dental tissues do not resemble teeth at all. This tumor commonly develops in younger dogs, less than 1 year of age and rarely in cats. On an intraoral radiograph, you will observe a defined mass of calcified material, which may be surrounded by a radiolucent band or a number of toothlike structures.[31] The recommended course of action is a wide excision to remove all affected tissue and teeth structures. Odontomas may be associated with a dentigerous cyst. A dentigerous or follicular cyst is a fluid-filled cyst surrounding the crown of an unerupted tooth, which can expand rapidly and cause destruction of bone. The recommended treatment is removal of the entire cyst lining along with any unerupted or partially erupted teeth to prevent the cyst from reoccurring.[31,33]

Gingival Hyperplasia

Gingival hyperplasia is a histological diagnosis and the condition may be more properly defined as a gingival overgrowth or enlargement. This type of oral tumor is presented in various degrees in dogs of any age, but more commonly seen in boxers and bulldogs (see web content: Figs. 7.50W–7.53W). These masses may mimic a neoplastic process and all should be charted, measured, and biopsied. An instrument that can be used to aid in removal of excessive tissue is the Goldman-Fox periodontal pocket marker. This probe is calibrated in increments of 2 mm and used to establish exterior puncture marks on the gingiva at the base of the pocket to help indicate the initial line of the incision. Gingival enlargement is commonly seen in dogs that are on a chronic regimen of cyclosporine, phenobarbital, or calcium channel blockers, such as amlodipine. Gingival enlargement is not as common in cats, but some cases have been seen in Maine coons, British shorthairs, and has been noted in kidney recipients that are on a long-standing dose of cyclosporine. Treatment is typically excision with a surgical blade. Bleeding needs to be controlled by means of digital pressure, gauze, or swabs coated with hemostatic solution. Cautery, radiosurgery, electrosurgery, a diamond bur, or laser therapy are options to remove large amounts of abnormal gingiva. A crown prep bur or 12-fluted bur may be used to contour the gingiva. Finally, a gingival dressing, consisting of a tincture of benzoin and myrrh is applied to the affected sites.[34]

Papillomas

Papillomas are benign oral tumors, viral or nonviral in origin, and are commonly located on the gingiva, lips, tongue, and/or palate (see web content: Fig. 7.54W).[31,33,34] These are tumors transmitted from dog to dog by direct contact and typically affect younger animals.[31] They vary in size, may be a single or in a clustered pattern, pink or white in color, and are located on stalks. Most papillomas resolve within several weeks, so removal is often unnecessary, unless there is trauma causing bleeding or difficulty eating.[31,33] If the papillomas are removed, they should be biopsied. It is common for these tumors to reoccur.

Eosinophilic Granulomas

Eosinophilic granulomas are another type of oral mass, seen more often in cats than in dogs (see web content: Fig. 7.55W).[31,33,34] However, several cases have been reported in cavalier King Charles spaniels. Severe ulcers or plaques may be located on the upper lip area, the tongue, palate, and glossopalatine arches. If the ulcers are significant, it could lead to anorexia and weight loss. Diagnosis is achieved with a biopsy, as lab work may or may not show eosinophilia.[31] Treatment consists of high-dose corticosteroid therapy, such as prednisone, to control the lesions. Another option may be the use of methylprednisolone acetate injection to control the lesions. Other therapies include flea control and feeding a hypoallergenic diet.[31]

Malignant Oral Tumors and Treatments

Malignant oral tumors may be both locally invasive and metastatic. The diagnostic plan is often the same for benign or malignant tumors.

Common malignant oral tumors found in dogs are malignant melanoma, squamous cell carcinoma (SCC), and fibrosarcoma. Common malignant tumors found in cats include SCC and fibrosarcoma.[31,32]

Malignant Melanomas

Malignant melanomas are frequently found in cocker spaniels, miniature poodles, and chow chows, commonly affecting older male dogs.[32] These rapidly growing, discrete masses may be seen as raised, ulcerated, pigmented masses located on the gingiva or buccal mucosa (see web content: Figs. 7.56W and 7.57W).[31,32] They may be amelanotic or nonpigmented, with a necrotic surface.[31,33] They are occasionally located on the palatal tissues. Malignant melanomas are highly invasive to the jaw bones. Metastasis is common, involving the regional lymph nodes and lungs.[31,32]

Squamous Cell Carcinoma

SCC is the most common malignant oral tumor in cats.[32,33] It is commonly located on the palate, rostral mandible, sublingual mucosa, and on the caudal maxilla and has a red, cauliflower-like, ulcerated appearance (see web content: Fig. 7.58W). This is a progressive, rapidly growing tumor that is locally invasive, especially to the jaw bones.[31] Lingual SCC is common in older dogs, especially poodles, Labradors, and Samoyeds.[32] Metastasis is rare in cats, but in dogs involves spread to regional lymph nodes and then the lungs. Tumors found in the caudal oral cavity are more likely to metastasize than tumors located elsewhere.[31,32] Cats that have feline leukemia virus (FeLV), feline immunodeficiency virus (FIV), and that wear flea collars may be predisposed to the development of SCCs.[33,34] In young dogs, papillary SCC is seen frequently. It is less aggressive than ordinary SCC, but still requires surgical intervention.[31] The prognosis of SCC in cats is considered poor due to the fact that it is locally invasive and often is not diagnosed until the tumor has spread.[31,33]

Fibrosarcomas

Fibrosarcomas are slow-growing tumors routinely found on the caudal maxilla and/or palate, appearing as firm, flat, diffuse masses.[32,33] Fibrosarcomas are more common in large-breed, middle-aged, male dogs.[31] They may be less commonly located on the mandible, but have been shown to deeply infiltrate the adjacent soft tissues and bone. Metastasis is uncommon.[31] In large-breed dogs, especially golden retrievers, a histologically benign but biologically aggressive fibrosarcoma exists, which may be misdiagnosed as a fibroma or other benign oral mass.[31–33]

Osteosarcoma

Osteosarcoma may involve the maxilla or mandible, but the primary tumor may be difficult to locate. It may not be seen without intraoral radiographs.

Treatments

The most recommended treatment for malignant tumors is surgical removal, with the goal being to remove the primary tumor with a margin of unaffected tissue to prevent recurrence.[32] The type of surgery will depend on the type and location of the primary tumor. Typical oral surgeries may include partial mandibulectomy, partial maxillectomy, tonsillectomy, and partial glossectomy. Surgery consists of surgical excision of the primary mass, the surrounding tissues, and lymph nodes.[31]

Clients often request a debulking of a tumor, perhaps in hopes of delaying the growth of the tumor or removing the visible portion that the pet may be traumatizing. "Debulking" or partial removal of the tumor is largely considered unrewarding because oral tumors tend to recur rapidly and may become more ulcerated once debulked. Surgical removal will prevent local recurrence, but is not adequate as monotherapy for tumors such as malignant melanoma, due to the high incidence of metastasis to the regional lymph nodes and the need to achieve 2 cm margins.[32] Surgery is often combined with chemotherapy and/or radiation therapy.[31,33]

No surgical procedure is without complications. Intraoperative complications to expect include blood loss and hypotension, which can be prevented and/or treated. Postoperatively, watch for incisional dehiscence, epistaxis, swelling, and self-trauma.[31–33] Patients, especially cats, may require the placement of a temporary feeding tube after major oral surgery.[31,33]

In some instances, chemotherapy will prolong a good quality of life by controlling metastasis in patients where surgery or radiation therapy have removed or controlled the local tumor.[33] Chemotherapy may be used in combination with surgery and radiation therapy in the treatment of highly metastatic tumors, such as malignant melanoma and tonsillar SCC.[31,32]

Radiation therapy is used to treat the primary tumor site if the tumor is expected to be radiation sensitive or if surgical margins are determined to be "dirty."[31,32] A "dirty margin" is when there is evidence of malignant cells in the tissues of the surgical site. A combination of radiation therapy and surgery may provide tumor control while maintaining good function and appearance.[31] Radiation therapy may provide relief from clinical symptoms, such as pain and bleeding. Side effects may include inflammation, hair loss, anorexia, and scar formation.[31,33] Full-course radiation involves low doses of radiation for a total of 12–16 doses, given three times a week for 4 weeks.[31,32] There are minimal side effects locally, but treatment may lead to tumors in the area due to radiation exposure. Malignant melanomas have been shown to be sensitive to large doses of radiation.[32] This is also a good alternative for unresectable tonsillar SCCs and acanthomatous ameloblastomas. Fibrosarcomas are typically resistant to radiation therapy.[31–33]

In cases where more aggressive or definitive treatment is not an option, palliative radiation may be recommended. Palliative radiation calls for lower dose radiation, given once a week for 4 weeks.

Alternative therapies for carcinomas include the use of piroxicam.[32,33] This cyclooxygenase-2 (COX-2) inhibitor may interfere with tumor proliferation.[31] The treatment is palliative, in hopes of slowing tumor growth and helping with pain relief. The dose is 0.3 mg/kg every 48 hours in cats and every 24 hours in dogs. This dose may induce partial remission in some canine patients. Side effects include renal failure in cats and gastrointestinal ulceration in dogs.

A commercial vaccine is available for use in dogs with malignant melanoma. The canine melanoma vaccine is manufactured by Merial under the name Oncept™. Although the vaccine will not prevent the growth of the primary tumor, it may help prevent metastasis, thus increasing survival times.[31,32] The vaccine is administered with a transdermal device, with the doses given intramuscularly at 2-week intervals, for a total of four doses. Boosters are recommended at 6-month intervals. The vaccine is only available through a veterinary oncologist.[32]

Charting and Preparation of Samples

The World Health Organization (WHO) has recommendations for the staging of oral tumors in dogs and cats. This involves a tumor, node, metastasis (TNM) system as well.[31–33,35]

- Stage 0: No visible tumor
- Stage I: Tumor <2 cm in diameter, no lymph node involvement
- Stage II: Tumor 2–4 cm in diameter, no lymph node involvement
- Stage III: Tumor >4 cm in diameter, and/or lymph node involvement
- Stage IV: Tumor of any size, distant metastatic disease
- T: Primary tumor
  - Tis: Preinvasive carcinoma
  - T0: No evidence of a tumor
  - T1: Tumor <2 cm
  - T2: Tumor 2–4 cm
  - T3: Tumor >4 cm
  - T3a: Without bone invasion
  - T3b: With bone invasion
- N: Regional lymph node
  - N0: No evidence of regional lymph node involvement
  - N1: Movable ipsilateral nodes
  - N2: Movable contralateral or bilateral nodes
  - N3: Fixed nodes
  - N3a: Nodes do not contain tumor
  - N3b: Nodes contain tumor
- M: Distant metastasis
  - M0: No evidence of distant metastasis
  - M1: Distant metastasis, including distant nodes

Tissue biopsy is the only way to get a definitive diagnosis of an oral tumor. Knowing the type of tumor will help the veterinarian make recommendations as to treatment and prognosis.[31] Biopsies should be performed within the oral cavity using a scalpel blade or biopsy punch.[32] If the mass appears to involve the bone, a bone tissue sample should be submitted as well. Impression smears may also prove helpful to send along with the preserved specimens. If a mass is biopsied and given a histopathological diagnosis of "undifferentiated tumor," it should be reevaluated by another pathologist, preferably one who is familiar with oral tumors.[32] It may be helpful to include digital radiographs and pictures.

The prevalence of oral tumors in the dog and cat makes this an important topic for veterinary technicians to be aware of. With the ever-changing modalities of treatment, it is important to keep abreast of all the current literature.

References

1. Harvey, CE. 2005. Management of periodontal disease: understanding the options. *Veterinary Clinics of North America: Small Animal Practice* 35:819–836.
2. Lobprise, H, Wiggs, R. 2000. Periodontal disease. In *The Veterinarian's Companion for Common Dental Procedures*. Lakewood, CO: AAHA Press, pp. 47–62.
3. Bellows, J. 2007. Periodontal disease: periodontitis. In *Blackwell's Five Minute Veterinary Consult Clinical Companion: Small Animal Dentistry* (ed. HB Lobprise). Ames, IA: Blackwell, pp. 172–180.
4. Bellows, J. 2004. Dental radiography. In *Small Animal Dental Equipment, Materials and Techniques: A Primer*. Ames, IA: Blackwell, pp. 63–103.
5. Holmstrom, S, Frost-Fitch, P, Eisner, E. 2004. Periodontal therapy and surgery. In *Veterinary Dental Techniques for the Small Animal Practitioner*, 3rd edn. Philadelphia, PA: Saunders, pp. 233–290.
6. Bellows, J. 2004. Periodontal equipment and techniques. In *Small Animal Dental Equipment, Materials and Techniques: A Primer*. Ames, IA: Blackwell, pp. 115–173.
7. Gorrel, C, Derbyshire, S. 2005. Tooth extraction. In *Veterinary Dentistry for the Nurse and Technician*. Edinburgh: Elsevier Butterworth-Heinemann, pp. 119–129.
8. Bellows, J. 2007. Oronasal fistula. In *Blackwell's Five Minute Veterinary Consult Clinical Companion: Small Animal Dentistry* (ed. HB Lobprise). Ames, IA: Blackwell, pp. 188–193.
9. Peak, R.M. 2013. Antibiotics in periodontal disease. In *Veterinary Periodontology* (ed. BA Niemiec). Ames, IA: Wiley Blackwell, pp. 186–189.
10. Cleland, WP. 2000. Nonsurgical periodontal therapy. *Clinical Techniques in Small Animal Practice* 15:221–225.
11. Hale, FA. 2003. The owner-animal-environment triad in the treatment of canine periodontal disease. *Journal of Veterinary Dentistry* 20:118–122.
12. Holmstrom, SE, Frost Finch, P, Eisner, ER. 2004. Dental records. In *Veterinary Dental Techniques for the Small Animal Practitioner*, 3rd edn. Philadelphia, PA: Saunders, pp. 31, 33.
13. Holmstrom, SE, Frost Finch, P, Eisner, ER. 2004. Endodontics. In *Veterinary Dental Techniques for the Small Animal Practitioner*, 3rd edn. Philadelphia, PA: Saunders, p. 353.

14. American Veterinary Dental College (AVDC). www.avdc.org.
15. Eisner, ER. 2005. *Bites, Breath and Benevolent Breeding: A Dog Breeder's Guide to Healthy Bites and Oral Health*, 5th edn. Self published (contact author: dog-2thdoc@gmail.com).
16. Holmstrom, S, Frost-Fitch, P, Eisner, E. 2004. Orthodontics. In *Veterinary Dental Techniques for the Small Animal Practitioner*, 3rd edn. Philadelphia, PA: Elsevier, pp. 499–558.
17. Hennet, PR, Harvey, CE. 1996. Craniofacial development and growth in the dog. *Journal of Veterinary Dentistry* 9:11–18.
18. Tutt, C. 2006. Malocclusions and normal occlusions. In *Small Animal Dentistry: A Manual of Techniques*. Oxford: Blackwell, pp. 239–268.
19. Bellows, J. 1999. *Atlas of Canine Dentistry: Malocclusions and Breed Standards*. Waltham, MA: Vernon.
20. Reiter, AM. 2008. *Orthodontics: diagnosis and treatment of malocclusions*. University of Pennsylvania School of Veterinary Medicine, Philadelphia.
21. Surgeon, TW. 2004. Case studies: orthodontics and other dental surprises. In *Proceedings: Western Veterinary Conference*.
22. Verhaert, L. 1999. A removable orthodontic device for the treatment of lingually displaced mandibular canine teeth in young dogs. *Journal of Veterinary Dentistry* 15:69–75.
23. Harasan, G. 2008. Maxillary and mandibular fractures. *Canadian Veterinary Journal* 48:819–820.
24. Verstraete, FJM. 2004. Maxillofacial fractures. In *Veterinary Dental Techniques for the Small Animal Practitioner*, 3rd edn. (eds. S Holmstrom, P Frost Fitch, E Eisner). Philadelphia, PA: Elsevier, pp. 559–600.
25. Marretta, SM. 2001. Jaw fracture management. In *Proceedings: Atlantic Coast Veterinary Conference*.
26. Verstraete, FJM, Lommer, MJ. 2012. *Oral and Maxillofacial Surgery in Dogs and Cats*. Edinburgh: Saunders.
27. Niemiec, B. 2010. *Small Animal Dental, Oral, and Maxillofacial Disease: A Color Handbook*. London: Manson.
28. Newton, CD, Nunamaker, DM. 1985. *Textbook of Small Animal Orthopaedics*. Philadelphia, PA: Lippincott.
29. Verstraete, FJM. 2002. Maxillofacial fractures. In *Textbook of Small Animal Surgery*, Vol. 1 (ed. DH Slatter). Philadelphia, PA: Saunders.
30. *Merriam Webster's Medical Desk Dictionary*. 1996.
31. Liptak, JM, Withrow, SJ. 2006. *Oral tumors. In Withrow and MacEwen's Small Animal Clinical Oncology*, 4th edn. Philadelphia, PA: Saunders.
32. Coyle, VJ, Garrett, LD. 2009. Finding and treating oral melanoma, squamous cell carcinoma, and fibrosarcoma in dogs. https://www.dvm360.com/view/finding-and-treating-oral-melanoma-squamous-cell-carcinoma-and-fibrosarcoma-dogs ().
33. Dhaliwal, RS, Kitchell, BE, Manfra Marretta, S. 1998. Part 1: oral tumors in dogs and cats: diagnosis and clinical signs. Part 2: prognosis and treatment. *Compendium* 20:1109–1119.
34. Lobprise, HB (editor). 2007. *Blackwell's Five Minute Veterinary Consult Clinical Companion: Small Animal Dentistry*, 4th edn. Ames, IA: Blackwell.
35. Hahn, KA, DeNicola, DB, Richardson, RC et al. 1994. Oral malignant melanoma: prognostic utility of an alternative staging system. *Journal of Small Animal Practice* 35:251–256.

Feline Dentistry

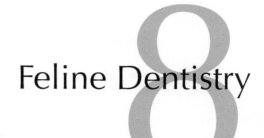

Jennifer Crawford, LVT, VTS (Dentistry) and
Billie Jean (Jeannie) Losey, RVT, VTS (Dentistry)

Learning Objectives

- Identify signs and symptoms of cats presenting with gingivostomatitis
  - State available treatments for cats presenting with gingivostomatitis
  - Identify causes of gingivostomatitis
  - State recommended diagnostics for cats presenting with gingivostomatitis
  - List the common medications used for treatment for cats presenting with gingivostomatitis
- Identify the three major forms of eosinophilic granuloma complex
  - Identify the possible causes of eosinophilic granuloma complex
  - State the prevalence of eosinophilic granuloma complex
  - Identify the symptoms of eosinophilic granuloma complex
  - Identify the commonly performed diagnostics for eosinophilic granuloma complex
  - Identify the different treatment options and drug dosages for treating eosinophilic granuloma complex
- Describe the pathogenesis of tooth resorption in cats
  - State the clinical signs and symptoms of tooth resorption in cats
  - Describe the stages, both clinically and radiographically, of tooth resorption in cats
  - State the diagnostics that are performed for tooth resorption in cats
  - State the dental charting abbreviations for tooth resorption in cats
  - Identify the treatment options for tooth resorption in cats

Small Animal Dental Procedures for Veterinary Technicians and Nurses, Second Edition.
Edited by Jeanne R. Perrone.
© 2021 John Wiley & Sons, Inc. Published 2021 by John Wiley & Sons, Inc.

Introduction

The objective for feline dentistry is to understand the unique dental conditions that our feline patients have. With some oral diseases, felines and canines are similar, but many of the diseases are slightly different and unique to felines. As discussed in Chapter 1, the differences in oral anatomy between canine and felines starts at the number of teeth. Felines are missing the maxillary first premolar and mandibular first and second premolars.

One disease that is similar in canine and feline patients is periodontal disease. The main difference is that in a feline the early stages of periodontal disease are visible after less of the periodontium has been destroyed. In a canine patient the normal sulcus depth is at 1–3 mm, whereas in a feline patient the normal is 0.5–1 mm. Another oral disease seen in both canines and the felines is oral neoplasia; squamous cell carcinoma is the most common type in felines.

In this chapter, we discuss the three oral diseases that are seen most commonly in our feline populations:

- Gingivostomatitis
- Eosinophilic granuloma complex
- Tooth resorption

The two most common oral conditions seen in our feline patients are tooth resorption and gingivostomatitis.[1] The third oral condition is eosinophilic granuloma complex, which may not be seen as often as tooth resorption and gingivostomatitis. Eosinophilic granuloma complex is common in the feline population and rare in the canine population.

Being able to identify these oral conditions will aid in producing a treatment plan. Having an understanding of these diseases will assist you in discussing the condition with your clients and help in giving comfort to the feline patient.

Gingivostomatitis

Jennifer Crawford, LVT, VTS (Dentistry)

This section aims to educate the technician in the oral condition gingivostomatitis. We will cover the recognition of the disease and the symptoms that may be noticed by the client, as well as the treatment options available.

Gingivostomatitis is a common and often a very debilitating oral disease in the feline. It can be described as an inflammation of the gingiva and the oral mucosa and is often a very painful condition (Fig. 8.1). There is no one exact cause for this condition, but there are many theories as to why it occurs and many ideas on how to treat. There are also many different terms associated with this disease, most of which are related to the cells that may be part of the cause (Table 8.1).

The most commonly accepted theory is that gingivostomatitis is an immune response or hypersensitivity to the plaque and bacteria that accumulate in the oral cavity. The immune system can be weakened or suppressed by many different agents,

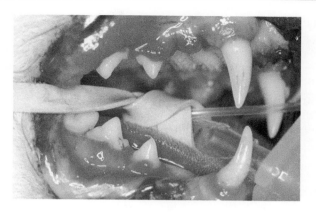

Figure 8.1   Presentation of stomatitis.

Table 8.1   Other names for gingivostomatitis

- Lymphoplasmacytic stomatitis (LPS)
- Lymphocytic plasmacytic gingivitis stomatitis (LPGS)
- Plasmacytic stomatitis (PS)
- Plasma cell gingivitis-stomatitis-pharyngitis
- Chronic ulcerative paradental stomatitis (CUPS)
- Necrotizing stomatitis
- Feline chronic gingivostomatitis
- Chronic gingivitis-stomatitis-faucitis

including viruses and bacteria, or without known cause. Viruses commonly associated with a suppressed immune system in cats include feline leukemia, feline immunodeficiency virus (FIV), and calicivirus. Another cause may be a bacterial component, such as bartonella, or there may be idiopathic reasons.

Symptoms of Gingivostomatitis

Gingivostomatitis can affect any feline breed, of either gender and at any age. Until recently, 2007, it was believed that certain breeds were more at risk, such as Persian, Abyssinians, Siamese, Himalayans, and Burmese.[2] Recent research has shown that the breed of cat does not play an important factor in the development of gingivostomatitis.[3]

There are a wide variety of symptoms associated with gingivostomatitis. The attached gingiva in a normal healthy cat is described as pink with a knifelike edge. In the early stages of gingivostomatitis, the edges appear to have a darker pink to red appearance and are slightly swollen. The appearance of the early stages of stomatitis can often mimic gingivitis, which makes follow-up care crucial for the patient. Halitosis is often associated with all stages of stomatitis, and as the disease progresses, the odor usually intensifies. The halitosis is associated with the bacterium that is building up on the teeth and at the gingival margins. Often, owners will notice an odor before noticing the inflammation in the oral cavity.

As the stomatitis progresses, it will be more apparent in the buccal gingival area. The gingiva will be bright red, with an ulcerated or swollen appearance. The caudal teeth (those behind the canine teeth) typically have more of the swollen, inflamed appearance as compared with the rostral teeth (the canine and incisor teeth) (Fig. 8.2). But that is not true in every case of gingivostomatitis (Fig. 8.3). The oral mucosa becomes very fragile and can spontaneously bleed upon palpation. Drooling is another common symptom that clients sometimes notice in a cat with any stage of gingivostomatitis. Anorexia may be linked with the advanced stages of gingivostomatitis but can be seen with any stage of the disease due to the pain and discomfort in the oral cavity. The ability to eat, drink, and even swallow may be affected for cats with any stage of stomatitis. It is common to see these cats wanting to eat or drink, but the pain and inflammation limit their ability to do so. The inability to swallow is severe when the cat's palatoglossal folds (formerly known as the fauces), the area between the pharynx and the oral cavity, are

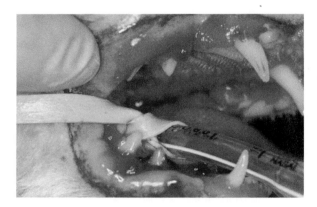

Figure 8.2   Presentation of stomatitis in the caudal mouth area.

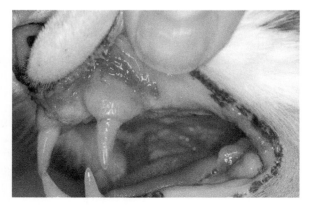

Figure 8.3   Presentation of stomatitis.

affected. Cats with gingivostomatitis can have any one or a combination of the above symptoms.

Diagnostics

A multitude of diagnostics can be performed to rule out other systemic disease that may need to be treated in addition to gingivostomatitis. The first and most important diagnostic tool is clinical observation by the client and by the practitioner, especially in the early stages of the disease when there are more treatment options available. A thorough physical exam should be performed, as well as a chemistry profile and a complete blood count. Often the serum total protein and serum globulins are elevated.[4] The viral status of feline leukemia and FIV should also be obtained, as oral stomatitis can be associated with these two diseases. Other viral and bacterial tests that can be performed are that for feline calicivirus and bartonella, as either of these can be linked to the onset or presence of stomatitis.[5]

Oral Evaluation

A thorough oral evaluation under anesthesia needs to be performed on the cat with gingivostomatitis, with the plaque, calculus, and gingival indexes being scored. The evaluation should grade each quadrant of the oral cavity, as each area may appear in different stages of the disease. Also, note the area of the palatoglossal folds that are affected. Photographs should be taken to document pretreatment and posttreatment; these will aid in the documentation of treatment progression. Photographs are also useful to give to the client, so they are aware of the severity of the disease. Intraoral radiographs are necessary in the evaluation process of cats affected with stomatitis to evaluate the root and bone structures (Figs. 8.4 and 8.5). As the disease progresses, the inflammation and destruction that occur with gingivostomatitis affect not only the gingival tissue but also the dental support structures such as the gingiva, periodontal ligament, and alveolar bone.

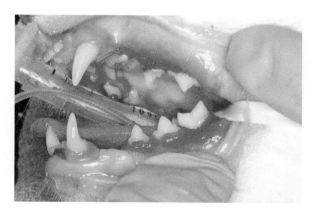

Figure 8.4   Presentation of stomatitis at the rostral area (canine tooth).

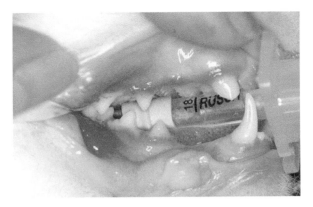

Figure 8.5   Right caudal mouth with stomatitis presenting tooth resorption (106, 107, 407) and bone loss (408) occurring along with stomatitis.

Frequently, tooth resorption on the roots can be found in addition to the ongoing stomatitis. It is important to assess the health of the tooth and periodontium to determine which treatment options will be best suited for the patient, either medical, surgical or a combination of both. Assessing the amount of support structure that has been destroyed by the disease will aid the practitioner in understanding how advanced the disease process is, and will help in deciding which treatment would be best suited for the patient.

A biopsy in the oral cavity may be recommended to confirm a diagnosis of gingivostomatitis and to rule out neoplasia. Many cancers, especially squamous cell carcinoma, can have a similar appearance in the early stages, but only a biopsy report can confirm the correct diagnosis.

Treatments

Gingivostomatitis can be a complicated oral disease to treat and usually will require a combination of medical and surgical treatments to make the patient more comfortable. A full dental cleaning consisting of supra- and subgingival cleaning and polishing needs to be performed before the start of either medical or surgical treatments.

Medical Management

Commonly, medical management does not give a long-term cure, but it can keep the patient comfortable. Medical management includes one or a combination of classes of medications, such as analgesics, antibacterials, anti-inflammatories, antivirals, immunosuppressants, and steroids (Table 8.2).

Pain management is an essential part of any therapy. Cats with stomatitis are commonly in pain and discomfort from the severe inflammation and irritation the condition causes in the oral cavity. Common medications used in pain management are butorphanol, fentanyl, tramadol, and buprenorphine. Nonsteroidal anti-inflammatory

Table 8.2   Common medications used to treat gingivostomatitis

Medication	Common dosage	Route of administration
Buprenorphine	0.01–0.03 mg/kg, every 6–8 hours	Transmucosal
Fentanyl	12.5 or 25 mcg/h, applied every 72–118 hours	Transdermal patch
Meloxicam	0.025 mg/kg	Injectable liquid or oral suspension
Methylprednisolone	20 mg, every 3–4 weeks	Injection
Clindamycin	11–33 mg/kg, every 24 hours	Oral tablet, capsule, or liquid
Amoxicillin/clavulanate	62.5 mg, every 12 hours	Oral tablet or suspension

drugs (NSAIDs) can help in controlling pain and inflammation, but because cats seem to have a high sensitivity to NSAIDs, long-term dosing must be used with caution. Buprenorphine and fentanyl are the easiest to give due to the method of delivery, either transmucosally or by delivery patch.

Antibacterials in the form of systemic medications and oral rinses can help in controlling oral bacteria. Common systemic medications are amoxicillin/clavulanate, clindamycin, doxycycline, and metronidazole. The most commonly used oral rinse is a chlorhexidine solution.

Herpes virus is known to cause oral inflammation. Antivirals such as lysine can be effective, in some measure, in stomatitis, but only if the herpes virus is known to be the cause.

Cats presenting with stomatitis show an active immune response to the inflammation occurring on the gingiva as well as to the bacteria in the plaque and saliva. That is why immunosuppressants can play a role in treating cats medically or in conjunction with surgical extractions. Many different immunosuppressants can be used, but the most common is cyclosporine. It has been shown to put 50% of cats into remission, while a higher percentage showed biased improvement.[3] As with many medications, close monitoring needs to be observed, and with cyclosporine, the cat's renal and hepatic values should be watched closely.

Steroids can be beneficial in treating stomatitis; prednisone tablets and methylprednisolone injections are the most commonly used. These medications are commonly used for their anti-inflammatory properties to help calm the gingiva. Steroids help with the inflammation and can give patients some relief for a limited time.

Surgical Treatment

Extraction is an option in the areas where there is inflammation. Some cat owners are hesitant to allow teeth to be extracted and want to continue the use of medications because they think that their pet would not be able to eat without teeth. Unfortunately, however, many patients become resistant to the drugs, and symptoms may return at a quicker pace. An additional concern with long-term use of medications is the continuation of inflammation after extraction of the affected teeth.

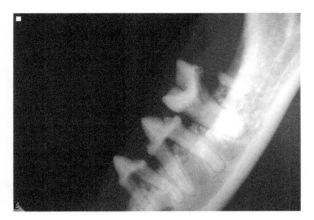

Figure 8.6   Radiograph to show tooth resorption and bone loss occurring along with stomatitis.

Extractions are the surgical treatment of choice. The number of teeth extracted depends on the severity of the case and the practitioner. Surgical treatment has shown to induce clinical remission of symptoms in some cases and is curative in others.[5] Surgical treatments need to be discussed when medical treatments have stopped providing benefits or if the client chooses not to go ahead with any medical management.

Laser surgery is also an option but may not be available in every area and is still a relatively new treatment option.[6] The goal of laser therapy is to remove the inflamed gingival tissue and to allow scar tissue to form. When the scar tissue forms in place of the gingival tissue, there is a decreased blood supply in the treated area, leading to a reduction in the immune response. Laser therapy does not always remove the need to treat in combination with medications and surgical extractions.

When discussing extractions, the number of extractions performed during one anesthetic period will be up to the practitioner. Each veterinarian has their own comfort level and ideas on how to perform these types of extraction cases. Most will choose to do caudal mouth extractions, which involve all the teeth behind the canines. They may also choose to perform extractions one side at a time or do only the most severely affected areas. The most important factor with these extractions is the removal of the entire tooth and root. If any part of the root is left in the socket, continued inflammation can occur. It is essential to use intraoral radiographs in order to check for retained root fragments (Fig. 8.6; see also web content: Figs. 8.7W and 8.8W).

A multimodal pain management protocol should be utilized when proceeding with extractions. Preoperative pain medication should be given to the patient to preempt the pain that the extractions will cause. Local and regional nerve blocks should also be used and applied to the areas to be addressed.

Aftercare

Postoperative care consists of pain medication that is easy for the client to give and the patient to consume. Postoperative feeding should consist of a soft canned diet that is easy for the cat to eat. If the cat is unable to eat due to pain, other alternatives must be discussed. Alternatives could include force-feeding, which would be difficult, especially if the cat is in pain and does not want the mouth to be handled, or placement of an esophagostomy tube, which would allow food and medications to be given directly into the esophagus. The placement of an esophagostomy tube would have to be discussed with the client before the procedure because placing the tube requires the patient to be under anesthesia. This procedure is best performed while the patient is undergoing extractions. Teaching around the use and care of the esophagostomy tube would need to be provided upon release. This tube would stay in for the recovery period of the patient, which will be from 1 to 2 weeks, or could be removed sooner if the cat can eat on its own without help.

In some cases, extractions are enough of a treatment to make the patient comfortable and functional. Many of these exceptions show a relation to the use of medications and the amount of time the patient had been managed with medications before surgical treatment.

Summary

The goal with our feline gingivostomatitis patients is to give them a quality life with as little pain as possible. Achieving this goal may require further medical management. As we have seen, there may not be a clear cause of this disease or treatment, but there are many ways to ensure the patient has a good quality of life.

Eosinophilic Granuloma Complex

Billie Jean (Jeannie) Losey, RVT, VTS (Dentistry)

Eosinophilic granuloma may be seen as an isolated lesion or part of the eosinophilic granuloma complex (see web content: Video 8.1W Eosinophilic granuloma complex). This complex includes three major forms:

- **Indolent ulcers:** These are typically seen as a well-circumscribed area on the upper lip, bilateral or unilateral with edges that are raised with superficial necrotic layers. These may occur at the philtrum of the upper lip or adjacent to the upper canine tooth.
- **Eosinophilic plaque** (not as common): This can be seen as a raised lesion or lesions that are yellowish to pink, moist, and commonly occur with miliary dermatitis and eosinophilic granuloma of the chin.
- **Eosinophilic granuloma:** This is seen as a single nodule or in groups that are linear and ulcerated. They can be found anywhere in the body, but most commonly on the abdominal region. These lesions can involve the oral mucosa, hard palate, soft palate, and the base of the tongue (causing dysphagia or ptyalism). Eosinophilic granuloma can be associated with halitosis, anorexia, and hypersalivation, and can be difficult to manage in the mouth.

Causes

The true cause of eosinophilic granuloma is unknown, but it could be caused by trauma and is also considered to be idiopathic in nature since the etiology is rarely determined. Most lesions are thought to be associated with chronic immune stimulation due to some underlying hypersensitivity, such as a food allergy, atopy, or insect allergy, in conjunction with a bacterial or viral infection. Eosinophilic ulcers have been associated with allergic responses to fleas and other allergens and trauma following a maxillary canine tooth extraction, which allows the mandibular canine to contact the upper lip.

Cats in the age range of 2–6 years old have a predisposition to eosinophilic granuloma complex, with females having twice the prevalence of males.[7] Eosinophilic plaque and eosinophilic granuloma may also have a genetic component.[7]

Symptoms

These lesions are mainly nonpainful but can be exacerbated on the tongue and lips due to licking. Patients present for anorexia and hypersalivation. On oral exam, lesions can be seen, which in more extensive cases may be ulcerated.[8]

Cats with larger lesions can have facial distortions. Indolent ulcers typically present unilaterally or bilaterally on the upper lips, with a circumscribed area of superficial necrotic layers with edges that are raised (Fig. 8.9).

Diagnostics

Diagnosis is primarily done with a physical exam, history, cytology, and/or histology. Biopsy is primarily used to exclude neoplasia and bacterial or viral aetiology,[9] and fungal infections.

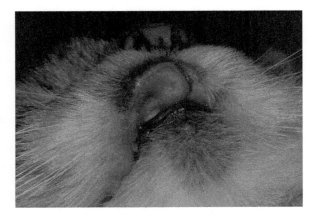

Figure 8.9   Example of an eosinophilic ulcer located on the maxillary lip of a cat (Courtesy of Dr. K.M. Murphy, North Carolina State University).

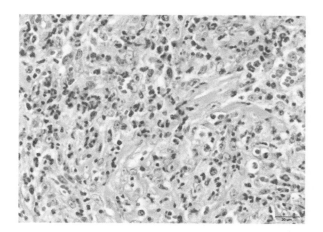

Figure 8.10 Histology sample of an indolent ulcer (Courtesy of Luke Borst, North Carolina State University).

A cytology sample can be taken by performing a scraping of the lesions. However, some irregular granulomas can grossly resemble squamous cell carcinoma and a biopsy would be needed to differentiate the two (Fig. 8.10).

Treatments

Medical Options

Due to the possible association with insect bite reaction and flea allergy, keeping the patient on a flea preventative and out of an insect environment is essential.

Antibiotics will sometimes have a therapeutic effect on the lesions, especially if there is a secondary bacterial infection. For eosinophilic/rodent ulcers, the choice of antibiotics are clindamycin 5.5 mg/kg twice a day orally, cephalexin 22 mg/kg orally every 12 hours, or amoxicillin trihydrate/clavulanate 12.5 mg/kg orally every 12 hours.[7]

Glucocorticoids, such as oral dexamethasone 0.1–0.2 mg/kg every 24 hours, can be used.[7] Since cats have fewer steroid receptors in their cells, they will need a higher dose than most species.[10] The higher dosage should be used as an induction dose but then tapered down as quickly as medically possible with a dose of 0.4 mg/kg orally every 24 hours. Injectable methylprednisolone acetate can be given at 4 mg/kg every 2 weeks as needed.[11] The dose for prednisone or prednisolone would range from 3 to 5 mg/kg every 24–48 hours orally.

Immunomodulation can be used for alternative therapy if the lesions are not responsive to steroid therapy. These drugs can include chlorambucil and levamisole.[11]

Surgery and Other Treatments

Surgery is an option for larger or single lesions that may need to be debulked in order for the patient to chew food more comfortably.

Other options that have been recommended are cryosurgery, laser therapy, and radiation therapies; these have been used with moderate success.[11]

Feline Tooth Resorption

Billie Jean (Jeannie) Losey, RVT, VTS (Dentistry)

Over the years, tooth resorption in cats has been given a variety of names. Some of the common names are feline odontoclastic resorptive lesions (FORLs), cervical line or neck lesion, and feline resorption or feline oral resorption. Neck lesion is a topographical distinction only. Inappropriate terms that are sometimes used include erosion or caries. In 2009, the term "tooth resorption" was officially adopted by the American Veterinary Dental College (AVDC) because the condition is recognized not only in felines but also in other species such as canines and primates (Figs. 8.11–8.13).

Definition and Symptoms

Tooth resorption is defined as the resorption of dental hard tissue by odontoclasts.[12] Odontoclasts are multinuclear cells that, when triggered, begin the resorption of primary deciduous teeth. Tooth resorption is the active resorption of the surface of the cementum by these cells (see web content: Video 8.2W Tooth resorption).

It was once believed these lesions were a result of periodontal disease, but the true cause is still unknown. This is a progressive disease and in stages 2, 3, and 4 it can be painful due to dentin and pulp exposure; however, it does not stop most patients from eating. The areas found to be most commonly affected are the mandibular third premolars, first molars, and the maxillary third and fourth premolars. Sometimes the lesion is confused with gingival hyperplasia. Once the lesion has started destroying enamel in the crown, granulation tissue will fill in the defect. The granulation tissue is often confused with gingival hyperplasia. Some common signs include the following:

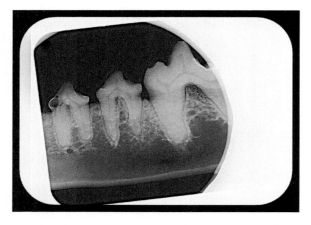

Figure 8.11   Radiograph of tooth resorption at #307 in a dog (Courtesy of William Krug, DVM, North Carolina State University).

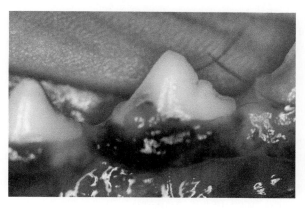

Figure 8.12 Photograph of tooth resorption in a premolar of a dog. Note the lesion at the gum line (Courtesy of William Krug, DVM, North Carolina State University).

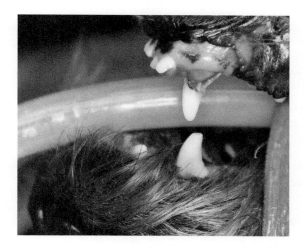

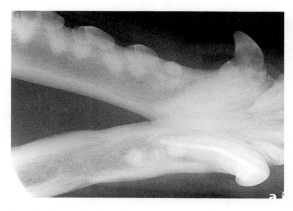

Figure 8.13 Photograph and radiograph of tooth resorption in a 5yr old canine patient of #404 with significant destruction starting at the cementoenamel junction.

CHAPTER 8

- Chattering of the jaw
- Dropping of food
- Hypersalivation
- Head shaking
- Sneezing
- Oral bleeding (related to inflammation of the gingival tissue)
- Anorexia (less common)

As the disease progresses, it moves coronally and the crown of the tooth may be lost. Clients may complain of missing teeth. As the resorption process advances through the crown and dentin, it exposes the tooth's pulp chamber to the oral cavity and oral bacteria.

There is no gender, breed, or age predisposition, but tooth resorption may develop at a younger age in purebred cats. Average age is 4–6 years.[12] Studies have shown that the percentage of mature cats that are clinically affected can be anywhere between 20% and 75%.[13]

Stages of Tooth Resorption

Tooth resorption is classified into five stages based on severity and into three types based on the location of the resorption.[13] Stages are defined by the AVDC as follows (Fig. 8.14):

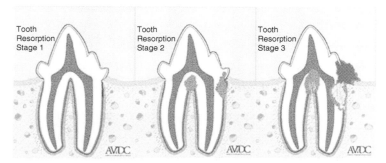

Tooth Resorption – AVDC Classification of Clinical Stages

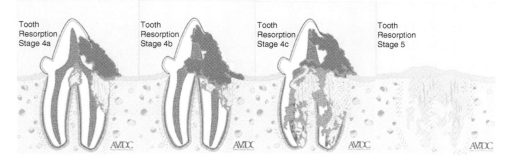

Figure 8.14   Diagram of tooth resorption stages in cats (Copyright AVDC, used with permission).

- Stage 1 (TR 1): Mild dental hard tissue loss. This is the hardest stage to identify[13,14]
- Stage 2 (TR 2): Moderate dental hard tissue loss[13,14] (Fig. 8.15)
- Stage 3 (TR 3): Deep dental hard tissue loss (extends into the pulp cavity). Most of the tooth retains its integrity[13,14] (Fig. 8.16)
- Stage 4 (TR 4): Extensive dental hard tissue loss. Most of the tooth has lost its integrity[13,14]
    - TR 4a: Crown and root are equally affected[13,14]
    - TR 4b: Crown is more affected than the root[13,14]
    - TR 4c: Root is more affected than the crown[13,14] (Fig. 8.17; see also web content: Fig. 8.18W)
- Stage 5 (TR 5): The crown is no longer visible; only ghost appearance of the hard tissue is visible on radiographs (see web content: Fig. 8.19W)[13,14]

Based on radiographic appearance, tooth resorption is then classified into three types: Treatment can be determined by the type of resorption.

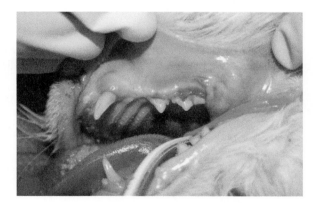

Figure 8.15   Stage 2 tooth resorption on #207 and #208. Notice that the enamel and part of the dentin are missing (Courtesy of William Krug, DVM, North Carolina State University).

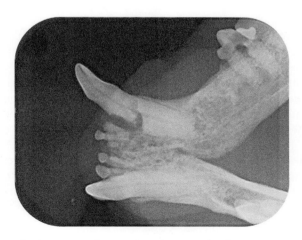

Figure 8.16   Radiograph of stage 3 tooth resorption (Courtesy of William Krug, DVM, North Carolina State University).

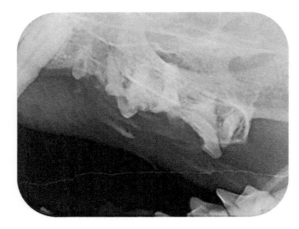

Figure 8.17   Stage 4a tooth resorption of #207 and stage 4b tooth resorption of #208; the crown is more affected (Courtesy of William Krug, DVM, North Carolina State University).

- ■ Type 1 (T1) tooth appearance: There is a focal or multifocal radiolucency, with otherwise normal radiopacity and a normal periodontal ligament space[13,14]
- ■ Type 2 (T2) tooth appearance: There is narrowing or disappearance of the periodontal ligament space in at least some areas and decreased radiopacity[13,14]
- ■ Type 3 (T3) tooth appearance: Types 1 and 2 appearance are included in the same tooth. The tooth has areas of normal and narrow or lost periodontal space. There is focal to multifocal areas of decreased radiolucency, and generalized decreased radiopacity in other areas of the tooth[13,14]

Diagnostics

Diagnosis of tooth resorption should be a combination of a thorough oral exam and intraoral radiographs. It is important to perform a thorough exam on all feline patients, especially since tooth resorption is so prevalent.[15] On oral exam on the awake patient, it may look as though part of the tooth's surface is missing or hyperplastic tissue is covering a portion of the tooth's crown. In some patients, the overlying gingiva or gingival margin will be severely inflamed, and in other areas, no inflammation is evident to indicate pathology is present.[13]

For the patient under anesthesia, each tooth should be evaluated with a periodontal probe and dental explorer. The explorer is used to detect pitted areas in the tooth's enamel and cementum by dropping down into the lesions. When the explorer is used correctly, it will make a "pinging" sound as it catches the edge of the lesion on its way out.

Caution is to be used at the mandibular molar due to its anatomy. The molar's furcation space can be misdiagnosed as a resorptive lesion. Intraoral radiographs should be taken; this will help you visualize if there is root resorption. No matter how insignificant a lesion may appear externally, there is always the potential for root resorption internally and externally.[16]

Charting

The abbreviation that is commonly used to note tooth resorption is TR. Once a stage has been determined, that stage number is recorded next to the abbreviation on the dental chart. On a tooth diagram, a dot is placed on the surface of the tooth with a circle around it to represent the location of the lesion and the dental radiographic charting abbreviations, for example TR3, added (see web content: Fig. 8.20W).

Charting tooth resorption on types based on radiographic appearance will include the stage plus the type. If you have a tooth that is in stage 3 and on radiograph there is a narrowing and disappearance of the periodontal ligament then we would assess the tooth as type 2 (see paragraph on "Stages of Tooth Resorption").

Treatment

The intraoral radiographs will determine treatment choices. Complete extraction of the tooth should always be attempted if no root resorption is noted and a normal periodontal ligament space is present on the dental radiograph.[7,13,15]

Crown amputation is a great treatment choice due to it being less invasive, making for an easier recovery for the patient; however, it can only be performed if no periodontal disease, endodontic disease, or gingivostomatitis is present.[15] A crown amputation is performed by making a small envelope flap and using a round bur or diamond round bur to cut the crown of the tooth off at the gingival margin. Once the crown of the affected tooth is removed, the roots and bone are smoothed down, and closure of the gingival flap is achieved with a 5-0 absorbable suture.[17] This treatment is only performed when root resorption is in the advanced stage as seen in a type 2 lesion, and no periodontal disease is present. Advanced stages are seen radiographically when the periodontal ligament is becoming difficult to distinguish from the surrounding alveolar bone, the roots, cementum, and dentin.

Dental radiographs are a very important tool when dealing with tooth resorption. Without this capability, it is not possible to properly stage and treat the lesion appropriately. Without properly staging these lesions, treating them could be done improperly and lead to more patient discomfort. If intraoral radiographs are not possible, refer these patients to a specialty practice that has dental radiographic capability (see web content: Fig. 8.21W).

Medical Options

Restorative procedures were once recommended in shallow lesions of stage 1 and some stage 2s to interrupt the progression of the lesion, provided that the roots look normal on radiographs.[16] But due to the progressive nature of the disease, it is no longer a recommended treatment. It was found (restorative treatment) to have a poor success rate – only 10–20% after a 2- to 3-year follow-up.[12] Oral applications of fluoride treatments have never been proven to help prevent or slow down the resorption process.

References

1. Girard, N, Servet, E, Biourge, V, Hennet, P. 2008. Feline tooth resorption in a colony of 109 cats. *Journal of Veterinary Dentistry* 25:166–174.
2. Wiggs, R, Lobprise, H. 1997. *Veterinary Dentistry: Principles and Practice*. Philadelphia, PA: Lippincott-Raven.
3. Ray, JD, Jordan, DG, Eubanks, DL, Crosswhite, ME. 2009. A review of stomatitis and treatment in cats. *International Journal of Pharmaceutical Compounding* 13:372–381.
4. Holmstrom, SE. 2000. Feline dentistry. In *Veterinary Dentistry for the Technician and Office Staff*. Philadelphia, PA: Saunders, p. 284.
5. Lyon, KF. 2005. Gingivostomatitis. *Veterinary Clinics of North America Small Animal Practice* 35:893.
6. Lewis, JR, Tsugawa, AJ, Reiter, AM. 2007. Use of CO_2 laser as an adjunctive treatment for caudal stomatitis in a cat. *Journal of Veterinary Dentistry* 24:240–249.
7. Bonello, D. 2007. Feline inflammatory, infectious and other oral conditions. In *BSAVA Manual of Canine and Feline Dentistry*, 3rd edn. (ed. C Tutt, J Deeprose, D Crossley). Gloucester: BSAVA, pp. 126–147.
8. Bellows, J. 2010. *Feline Dentistry: Oral Assessment, Treatment and Preventative Care*. Ames, IA: Wiley-Blackwell.
9. Buckley, L, Nuttall, T. 2012. Feline eosinophilic granuloma complex(ities): some clinical clarification. *Journal of Feline Medicine and Surgery* 14:471–481.
10. Werner, A. 2007. Eosinophilic granulomas. In *Blackwell's Five-Minute Veterinary Consult Clinical Companion, Small Animal Dentistry* (ed. HB Lobprise). Ames, IA: Blackwell, pp. 352–357.
11. White, S. 2010. Eosinophilic granuloma complex. In *The Merck Veterinary Manual* (ed. S Kahn). Whitehouse, NJ: Merck Sharp & Dohme, pp. 884–885.
12. Reiter, AM. 2007. Tooth resorption: feline. In *Blackwell's Five-Minute Veterinary Consult Clinical Companion, Small Animal Dentistry* (ed. HB Lobprise). Ames, IA: Blackwell, pp. 305–313.
13. Bellows, J. 2010. *Feline Dentistry: Oral Assessment, Treatment and Preventive Care*. Ames, IA: Wiley-Blackwell, pp. 120–126, 222–241.
14. American Veterinary Dental College. 2009. Tooth resorption. https://avdc.org/avdc-nomenclature/ (accessed March, 2020).
15. Niemic, BA. 2010. *Small Animal Dental, Oral and Maxillofacial Disease*. London: Manson Publishing, pp. 136–139.
16. Lobprise, H, Wiggs, R. 2000. *The Veterinarian's Companion for Common Dental Procedures*. Lakewood, CO: AAHA Press, pp. 143–146.
17. Niemiec, BA. 2008. Oral pathology. *Topics in Companion Animal Medicine* 23:59–71.

CHAPTER 8

Dentistry and the Exotic Patient

Kathy Istace, CVT, VTS (Dentistry)

Learning Objectives

- Identify the dental and oral anatomy in rodents, rabbits, ferrets, and other popular small exotic pets
- Recognize important differences between the dentition of the species mentioned above
- Describe commonly seen dental problems
- Become familiar with specialized dental instruments for exotic species
- Describe husbandry and home care for healthy mouths
- Learn about dental radiography in exotics

Small Animal Dental Procedures for Veterinary Technicians and Nurses, Second Edition.
Edited by Jeanne R. Perrone.
© 2021 John Wiley & Sons, Inc. Published 2021 by John Wiley & Sons, Inc.

Challenges of Exotic Dentistry

The species addressed in this section are rodents, rabbits, ferrets, and other popular small exotic pets. Anesthesia and pain management for exotic species could (and do!) have entire textbooks devoted to them, so the scope of this section will be limited to that for dental procedures.

Exotic caged pets are seen by many small animal veterinary practices, although in most practices, they are not dealt with as commonly as dogs and cats. Owners may also handle their smaller caged pets infrequently. This leads to two main difficulties when they are presented for dental treatment: that veterinary staff may not be as familiar with their dental diseases and appropriate treatment, anesthesia, and pain management; and that by the time the client notices a problem and the exotic patient is presented, it may be quite debilitated.

Rodent Dentistry

All rodents possess two pairs of continuously growing incisors and no canine teeth.[1] Rodents also lack a set of exfoliating primary teeth, growing only permanent teeth. However, not all rodents are created equal when it comes to the rest of their dentition. Two types of rodents will be discussed within this section: caviomorph rodents and murine rodents.

Caviomorph Rodents (Guinea Pigs, Chinchillas, Degus)

All teeth of caviomorph rodents have open root apices, allowing the teeth to grow continuously; this is a type of dentition called elodont.[2] Worn down by a diet of abrasive grasses and vegetation, the teeth are constantly replaced by new growth.

Oral Anatomy and Dentition of Caviomorph Rodents

$$2(I1/1, C0/0, P1/1, M3/3) = 20$$

The caviomorph oral cavity is small and narrow, with a large space, the diastema, separating the incisors from the cheek teeth.[3] The enamel on the incisor teeth is thickest on the facial surface and is a yellow-orange color. This pigmentation is not present in guinea pigs.[4] The cheek teeth have large chewing surfaces, and rather than being set parallel in the mouth, diverge caudally (Figs. 9.1–9.4; see web content: Chart 9.1W Chinchilla Dental Assessment Chart and Chart 9.2W Guinea Pig Dental Assessment Chart).

Murine Rodents (Rats, Mice, Hamsters, Gerbils)

Murine rodents possess continuously growing incisors that allow them to nest and to tunnel through hard obstacles to gain access to food, but they do not have continuously growing cheek teeth.[4] Murines consume diets of seeds, roots, and tubers,

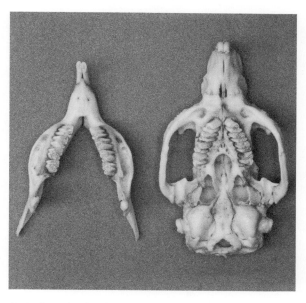

Figure 9.1   Guinea pig skull: occlusal surfaces (Courtesy of Skulls Unlimited International Inc.).

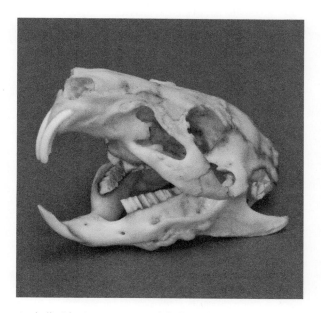

Figure 9.2   Guinea pig skull: side view (Courtesy of Skulls Unlimited International Inc.).

which are not particularly abrasive. Their molars possess true anatomical roots and short crowns, called brachyodont.[4]

Oral Anatomy and Dentition of Murine Rodents

$$2\left(I1/1, C0/0, P0/0, M3/3\right) = 16$$

CHAPTER 9

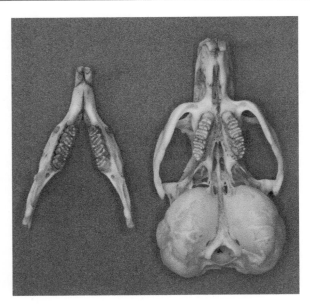

Figure 9.3 Chinchilla skull: occlusal surfaces (Courtesy of Skulls Unlimited International Inc.).

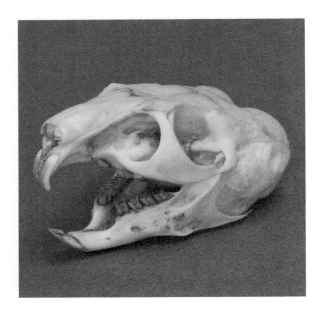

Figure 9.4 Chinchilla skull: side view (Courtesy of Skulls Unlimited International Inc.).

Murine rodents possess the same sort of long, narrow oral cavity as caviomorph rodents; however, cheek tissue fills the diastema between the incisors and the molars.[4] Hamsters have large cheek pouches that are used to store and carry food, bedding, and their young. As with all rodents, murines have two pairs of elodont incisors. The mandibular incisors are normally three times longer than the maxillary incisors.[5] The enamel is thicker on the facial surface of the incisors and is orange in color.

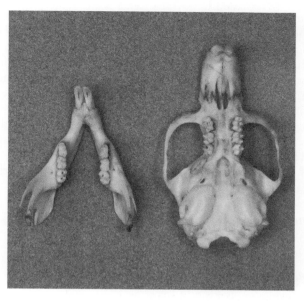

Figure 9.5 Hamster skull: occlusal surfaces (Courtesy of Skulls Unlimited International Inc.).

There are no canine teeth or premolars. The molars are brachyodont and situated caudally in the mouth (Fig. 9.5; see also web content: Fig. 9.6W and Chart 9.3W Rat, Mouse, Hamster Dental Assessment Chart).

Oral Examination of Rodents

The face and head should be first assessed for any asymmetry, swellings, ocular or nasal discharge, drooling, saliva staining, inability to close the mouth, obvious incisor overgrowth, and/or abnormal incisor wear pattern. A complete intraoral examination of the awake rodent is difficult. An otoscope can sometimes be used in larger awake rodents to visualize the oral cavity and cheek teeth, but more often, the pet will need to be sedated or anesthetized.[6] Mouth gags, cheek dilators, magnifiers, and dental mirrors can be used in the sedated/anesthetized patient to improve visualization of the caudal oral cavity. Check for an unlevel occlusal plane, sharp points or hooks on the cheek teeth, food impaction between teeth, tongue entrapment, soft tissue lacerations or ulcerations, cheek pouch impaction, stomatitis, or fractured teeth (see web content: Figs. 9.7W–9.9W). Skull radiographs should also be obtained as part of the complete oral examination; these allow occlusal evaluation and can reveal tooth root elongation and periapical lucencies.[7]

Anesthesia and Pain Management

Preanesthetic fasting should be limited to 1 hour, as these small patients do not vomit and are at risk of developing hypoglycemia.[8] Preanesthetic blood panels should be run on those patients large enough for venipuncture. The lateral saphenous or cephalic veins are the most accessible to collect small amounts of blood and for intravenous catheter placement (use 24 gauge or smaller) for emergency access with or without fluid administration.

Some procedures, such as oral examinations or incisor trimming, can be done using only chemical restraint. Drugs such as ketamine, oxymorphone, butorphanol, midazolam, medetomidine, glycopyrrolate, and atropine are commonly used to provide sedation, reduce the stress associated with induction, decrease salivary secretions, and provide pain relief. There are many excellent texts and resources that can be consulted with regard to rodent drug protocols and dosages[8] (Table 9.1).

Intubation of very small rodents is generally not an option. Alternately, a kitten-sized anesthetic mask on a nonrebreathing system can be used to induce anesthesia with isoflurane and O_2 administration. Anesthetic maintenance can be accomplished by placing a small anesthetic mask over only the nose, or by using a rubber catheter thin enough to fit into a nostril cut to accept an endotracheal tube adapter and trimmed to extend approximately 1 inch (25 mm) into one of the nostrils while the other nostril is occluded by a finger.[1] For murines, chamber induction can be used. A large anesthetic mask placed over the patient with the mask's diaphragm pressed firmly against a table can serve as a makeshift induction chamber. For anesthetic maintenance, a rubber dental dam or the palm of an examination glove is stretched over the end of a Bain system anesthetic hose using an elastic band to keep it in place. The patient's nose is placed through an "X" cut in the rubber, leaving the mouth free. A staff member must hold the nasal tube or mask to keep it in place. This person can also be dedicated to anesthetic monitoring

Table 9.1   Some common drugs and dosages for premedication of rodents and other small exotic pets

Agent	Guinea pig	Chinchilla	Hamster	Rat/mouse	Hedgehog	Sugar glider
Ketamine	5–40 mg/kg SC, IM, IV	5–40 mg/kg SC, IM, IV	50–100 mg/kg IM	22–44 mg/kg IM	5–20 mg/kg IM	20 mg/kg IM
Oxymorphone	0.2–0.5 mg/kg SC, IM	0.2–0.5 mg/kg SC, IM	0.2–0.5 mg/kg SC, IM	0.2–1.5 mg/kg SC, IM	–	–
Butorphanol	0.2–2.0 mg/kg SC, IM	0.2–2.0 mg/kg SC, IM	1–5 mg/kg SC	0.2–2 mg/kg SC	0.05–0.4 mg/kg SC	0.1–0.5 mg/kg SC, IM
Midazolam	1–2 mg/kg SC, IM, IV	1–2 mg/kg SC, IM, IV	1–2 mg/kg IM	1–2.5 mg/kg SC, IM	0.25–0.5 mg/kg IM	0.25–0.5 mg/kg IM
Medetomidine	0.3 mg/kg SC, IM	–	0.1 mg/kg SC	0.03–0.1 mg/kg SC	0.1 mg/kg IM	–
Glycopyrrolate	0.01–0.02 mg/kg SC	0.01–0.02 mg/kg SC	0.01–0.02 mg/kg SC	0.01–0.02 mg/kg SC	–	0.01–0.02 mg/kg SC, IM, IV
Atropine	0.05–0.2 mg/kg SC, IM, IV	0.05–0.2 mg/kg SC, IM, IV	0.04–0.4 mg/kg SC, IM	0.05–0.4 mg/kg SC, IM	0.01–0.04 mg/kg SC, IM	0.01–0.02 mg/kg SC, IM

IM, intramuscular; SC, subcutaneous; IV, intravenous.
Source: Adapted from Morrisey and Carpenter.[8]

(see web content: Fig. 9.10W). Heart rate can be monitored via pediatric stetho- scope, Doppler blood pressure monitor (Doppler crystal can be held or taped directly over the fur of the chest in most patients), or a lingual SpO_2 sensor placed on a foot, ear, or scrotum. Visualization of the mucous membrane color (tongue is especially useful) and the chest movements of respirations is essential. Circulating warm water blankets, microwavable oat bags (see web content: Fig. 9.11W), and exam gloves filled with warm water can all be useful in maintaining body temperature.

Small mammals do not often show obvious signs of pain, but this does not mean they should be denied pain relief.[6] Pain management can include narcotics used in premedication, injectable analgesics such as buprenorphine, and oral nonsteroidal anti-inflammatory drugs (NSAIDs) such as meloxicam. The placement of dental local blocks in rodents is usually impossible. Some signs that pain relief is not adequate are teeth grinding, hiding, depression, and anorexia. Pain must be recognized and treated quickly as rodents can become debilitated very quickly if not eating.

Common Dental Problems of Rodents

Malocclusion

The most common dental problem seen in rodents is malocclusion, causing overgrowth of the incisors (with or without cheek teeth in caviomorphs)[1] (see web content: Fig. 9.12W). Secondary tongue entrapment, in which the lower cheek teeth overgrow and due to their angulation arch over the tongue, preventing the animal from prehending food or swallowing; soft tissue lacerations of the tongue and buccal mucosa; tooth root elongation; and excess salivation ("slobbers") can occur. Malocclusions can result from traumatic injury to a tooth causing a loss of a portion of the crown and subsequently the loss of normal wear on the opposing tooth, or can result from hereditary conditions such as a mandible that is too narrow or too short, nutritional deficiencies such as not consuming enough roughage resulting in insufficient tooth wear, weakness of the jaw muscles, or behavioral problems such as cage chewing (see web content: Fig. 9.13W).

Treatment

Traumatic malocclusions are treated by smoothing the edges of the fractured tooth with a bur or file to reduce soft tissue injuries, treating the pulp if exposed by removing any infected tissue and capping it with calcium hydroxide paste topped with a thin layer of glass ionomer, and performing routine odontoplasty (also referred to as crown height reduction or occlusal leveling) on the opposing tooth until the fractured tooth regrows.[1] Atraumatic malocclusions can be treated, although not usually cured, with routine odontoplasty (usually every 6–8 weeks for the remainder of the animal's life), extraction of the affected teeth, dietary changes, or reducing the animal's stressors in cases of behavioral problems such as cage chewing or barbering. For details of odontoplasty and extraction, see the "Rabbit Dentistry" section (see web content: Figs. 9.14W and 9.15W).

Tooth Root Abscess

Tooth root abscess can be secondary to infection due to food or debris impaction between teeth, which spreads periapically,[1] tooth fracture leading to endodontic disease, or plaque-associated periodontal disease.[1,7] Facial swelling is the most common presentation.[1] Radiographs are necessary to determine whether the abscess is from the teeth and, if so, from which tooth. The location of facial swelling can be misleading, as the root apex of the incisors can extend to the premolars in caviomorphs and beyond the third molar in murine rodents. Tooth root abscesses of elodont teeth are usually very difficult to resolve, possibly due to the difficulty of completely removing all abscess material. They often require multiple procedures for extraction of the affected teeth, surgical debridement of the abscess, long-term antibiotic administration, and possible force-feeding.[7] Abscessed brachyodont teeth may be extracted using a small luxator or an 18 gauge needle. Suturing the gingiva closed over the extraction sites is very difficult in these tiny patients, so they are usually left open to heal.

Scurvy

Like humans, guinea pigs cannot synthesize vitamin C from glucose, and so require vitamin C supplementation from their diet. If vitamin C is not provided or ingested, they will develop scurvy. Oral signs of scurvy include gingival bleeding and loose teeth, sometimes resulting in malocclusion.

Cheek Pouch Impaction and Eversion

The cheek pouches of hamsters can become impacted if sticky, dry, or sharp materials are ingested and the hamster is unable to remove these materials from the pouch. The impacted pouch needs to be emptied and rinsed clean with saline. Long-term impaction can lead to stomatitis, and oral antibiotics may be necessary.[1]

Cheek pouches may also become everted, appearing as a pink, moist mass protruding from the mouth. The pouch should be replaced and a suture placed through the cheek to prevent re-eversion (see web content: Fig. 9.16W).

Caries and Tooth Resorption

Feeding a diet high in sugars or refined carbohydrates can cause dental caries in rodents. Tooth resorption can also occur, possibly secondary to periodontal inflammation.[1] Extraction is the treatment of choice for brachyodont teeth, or for elodont teeth that have extensive damage.[6] If a carious lesion is present on an elodont tooth that otherwise appears healthy and is still erupting, odontoplasty (and pulp capping if necessary) can be attempted.

Periodontal Disease

Plaque-induced periodontal disease can affect brachyodont teeth, particularly in pet rats.[7] These patients should have dental prophylaxis and extraction of teeth that have advanced attachment loss or infection. Periodontal disease involving elodont teeth is much more likely to be due to impaction of food or debris.

Dental Instruments

A complete set of rodent dental instruments comprises a mouth gag and cheek dilators to ensure adequate visualization of the oral cavity, and a rodent tongue depressor to protect the tongue and soft tissues of the mouth from trauma. High-speed burs (e.g., FG330, FG701) are used for incisor trimming, and low-speed burs (e.g., HP5, HP8, HP558) and/or molar/premolar rasps are used for crown height reduction of overgrown premolars and molars. A pair of rodent molar/premolar cutters can be used if no drill is available. For extraction of elodont teeth, a set of incisor and molar/premolar luxators are required, which are inserted into the periodontal space lateral to the tooth being extracted, then held while applying pressure longitudinally for 20 seconds. This is then done on the mesial aspect of the tooth being extracted, and the process repeated until the periodontal ligament is torn and the tooth is mobile. Extraction forceps are then used to intrude the tooth into the alveolar socket in a rocking motion to tear any remaining periodontal ligament and damage the apical germinal tissue to prevent tooth regrowth. Lastly, the extraction forceps are used to extract the tooth completely.[7]

Other useful tools include magnifying loupes, 18 gauge needles to luxate very small teeth, a saliva ejector suction tip fitted with a urinary catheter to suction fluid and debris from the mouth, and cotton-tipped applicators to staunch blood flow, absorb fluid, and remove debris from the mouth.

Husbandry and Home Care

Debilitated patients or patients who have had oral surgery may need nutritional support. A variety of soft foods can be offered or force-fed, such as Oxbow Critical Care (Oxbow Animal Health, Murdoch, NE; www.oxbowanimalhealth.com), which is a recovery food in powder form that is mixed with water and fed from a syringe; yogurt; or hay, vegetables and water pureed in a blender. Abscess-flushing syringes with the tips trimmed off halfway work to force-feed chinchillas and guinea pigs, and 1–3 mL syringes work well for tinier patients (see web content: Fig. 9.17W). Distasteful medications such as enrofloxacin may be mixed with apple juice or other juices in the dosing syringe to improve palatability.

To aid in preventing dietary-related malocclusions, owners should feed caviomorph rodents the majority of their diets as roughage, such as timothy hay, fresh greens, and vegetables. At most, one-third of their diets should consist of commercial pellets. Guinea pigs must also be given vitamin C supplementation to prevent scurvy. Stress can often be reduced by enlarging the animal's cage, removing or adding companions, or adding stimulation such as toys and mazes. Chew aids, such as wooden blocks, can help wear down rodent incisors.

Miscellaneous Small Pets

Hedgehogs

$$2(I2 - 3 / 2, C1 / 1, P3 - 4 / 2 - 3, M3 / 3) = 34 - 40$$

The hedgehog is an insectivore and has an oral anatomy that is quite different from that of other exotic pets. Anatomical characteristics of insectivores include small, long, narrow snouts, and a primitive tooth structure. The teeth of hedgehogs have true anatomical roots and do not grow continuously.[9] Hedgehogs possess deciduous teeth, which are replaced by permanent dentition beginning at 7–9 weeks of age. The incisors are used as forceps for picking up small prey, and the canines often resemble incisors or first premolars (see web content: Figs. 9.18W and 9.19W).

Complete oral examination of a hedgehog requires anesthesia or chemical restraint because of their self-protective behavior of rolling into a tight ball when stressed.

Hedgehogs are known to develop periodontal disease[9] (see web content: Fig. 9.20W). Owners will often present their hedgehogs because they have noticed a bad smell associated with the pet and/or inappetance. Treatment involves antibiotics, supportive care by force-feeding anorectic patients, and extraction of the diseased teeth (see web content: Fig. 9.21W).

Sugar Gliders

$$2(I3 / 2, C1 / 0, P3 / 3, M4 / 4) = 40$$

Sugar gliders are small nocturnal marsupials native to Australia and New Guinea that feed on insects and tree sap, although in captivity they are generally fed commercial pellets, proteins such as pinkie mice, mealworms, eggs, or cooked chicken, along with fruits and vegetables. Anesthesia is usually necessary for a complete oral examination, although restraint and examination while awake can be attempted in the morning, when they are more inactive. Their lower incisors are designed for stripping the bark from trees.[10] (see web content: Figs. 9.22W and 9.23W). All of their teeth have true anatomical roots and do not grow continuously. Periodontal disease can occur in gliders fed large amounts of soft carbohydrates. Teeth can also fracture from chewing sticks or cage wires. Dental prophylaxis and antibiotic therapy are recommended, although extraction of diseased teeth, especially of the long mandibular incisors, may risk jaw fracture.

Rabbit Dentistry

Rabbits belong to the order Lagomorpha. All teeth in lagomorphs have no true anatomical roots and grow continually, a type of dentition called elodont. Deciduous teeth are replaced by permanent teeth by 5 weeks of age.[7]

Oral Anatomy and Dentition of Rabbits

$$2(I2/1, C0/0, P3/2, M3/3) = 28$$

The oral cavities of rabbits are long and narrow, with a large space, the diastema, separating the incisors from the cheek teeth. The oral cavity is further divided by buccal skin folds halfway along the diastema.[11] Prehension of food is performed by the lips, tongue, and incisors in the rostral cavity. The actual chewing of food is done by the ridged cheek teeth in the caudal oral cavity. The mandible is narrower than the maxilla. Lagomorphs have four maxillary incisors – two anterior and two posterior.[12] The posterior incisors are smaller than the anterior ones and are commonly referred to as "peg" teeth (Figs. 9.24 and 9.25).

Oral Examination of Rabbits

The face and head should be first assessed for asymmetry, swellings, ocular or nasal discharge, drooling or wet fur, saliva staining, hair loss, obvious incisor overgrowth, and/or abnormal incisor wear pattern. A thorough oral examination is difficult in the awake rabbit because the long and narrow oral cavity allows only the anterior portion of the mouth to be readily visualized, and often there is food within the mouth that may obscure the teeth. An otoscope may be used to look into the oral cavity of the awake patient, but as few as 50% of problems can be recognized this way.[11] Sedation or general anesthesia will allow mouth gags, cheek dilators, magnifiers, and dental mirrors to be used to improve visualization of the caudal oral cavity (Fig. 9.26). Look and feel for an unlevel occlusal plane, sharp points on the teeth,

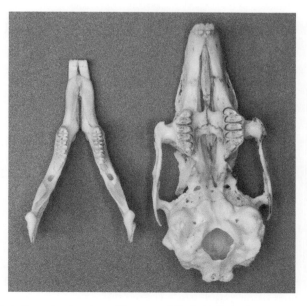

Figure 9.24   Rabbit skull: occlusal surfaces (Courtesy of Skulls Unlimited International Inc.).

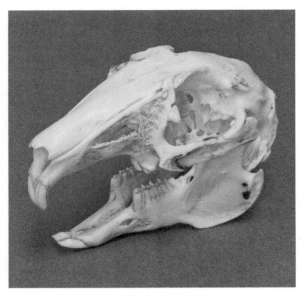

Figure 9.25   Rabbit skull: side view (Courtesy of Skulls Unlimited International Inc.).

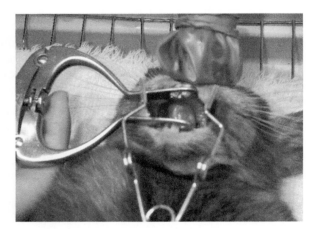

Figure 9.26   Rabbit with mouth gag and cheek dilators in place.

food impaction between teeth, soft tissue lacerations, tooth mobility, or fractured teeth. Skull radiographs are necessary to reveal tooth root elongation and periapical lucencies (see web content: Chart 9.4W Rabbit Dental Assessment Chart).

Anesthesia and Pain Management

Preanesthetic fasting may cause hypoglycemia and intestinal ileus in rabbits, and rabbits cannot vomit, increasing the risk of aspiration pneumonia. Fasting should be limited to 0–4 hours prior to sedation to allow the pet to clear any food content from its mouth.[13] As a minimum, packed cell volume and total protein (PCV/TP) and blood glucose should be measured. The cephalic veins, lateral saphenous, or the marginal ear vein are the most accessible to collect small amounts of blood and for intravenous catheter placement for emergency access with or without fluid administration.

Sedation or anesthesia in the debilitated rabbit is risky, so patients should be given antibiotics, pain relief, force-feeding, and so on as necessary to correct any preexisting conditions before attempting anesthesia.

Some procedures, such as oral examinations or incisor trimming, can be done using only chemical restraint. Drugs such as ketamine, midazolam, medetomidine, buprenorphine, butorphanol, and glycopyrrolate are commonly used to provide sedation, reduce the stress associated with anesthetic induction, decrease salivary secretions, and provide pain relief. There are many excellent texts and resources that can be consulted with regard to rodent drug protocols and dosages[8,13] (Table 9.2).

Due to the small oral cavity, large tongue, and caudal location of the glottis, intubation of rabbits can be difficult. It is easy to traumatize the trachea during repeated intubation attempts. The rabbit is first masked down with isoflurane or sevoflurane, or alternatively general anesthesia can be induced with intravenous drugs such as propofol, or ketamine and diazepam. Two types of intubation can then be attempted: direct visualization or blind intubation.[13] In either case, the rabbit is anesthetized by intravenous or inhalant agents, and is placed in sternal recumbency with the head and neck hyperextended. A 2.0–3.5 mm endotracheal tube is used with local anesthetic gel applied to the end to ease intubation. In direct intubation, the tongue is grasped and pulled to the side. Gauze ties placed around the upper and lower incisors can be used to open the mouth as wide as possible. A laryngoscope is inserted into the mouth so that the glottis is visualized, and the endotracheal tube is slid down the blade of the laryngoscope and into the trachea. For blind intubation, the rabbit must be breathing on its own as this technique requires respiratory noise to allow the operator to guide the tube into the correct position. The endotracheal tube is passed over the base of the tongue and the tube is advanced while listening for respiratory noise at the adapter end of the tube. If respiratory noise is not heard and the rabbit is breathing, the tube has entered the esophagus. If respiratory noise

Table 9.2   Common drug dosages for rabbit dentistry

Use	Agent	Dosage
Premedication	Ketamine	5–50 mg/kg IM, IV
	Midazolam	0.25–2 mg/kg IM
	Dexmedetomidine	0.05–0.125 mg/kg IM
	Glycopyrrolate	0.01–0.02 mg/kg IM, SC, IV
Anesthesia	Propofol	3–6 mg/kg IV
	Ketamine/diazepam	20–25 mg/kg (K)/1–5 mg/kg (D) IV
Analgesia	Buprenorphine	0.01–0.05 mg/kg IM, SC, IV
	Butorphanol	0.2–2.0 mg/kg IM, SC
	Meloxicam	0.1–0.3 mg/kg SC, PO
	Carprofen	1.5–5.0 mg/kg SC, PO

IM, intramuscular; SC, subcutaneous; IV, intravenous; PO, per os.
Source: Adapted from Hawkins and Pascoe.[13]

becomes louder, the tube is still on its way to entering the trachea. Once the tube is fully advanced and respiratory noise is still heard, the rabbit has been successfully intubated.

Another option for intubation in rabbits is an endotracheal tube called the v-gel®, manufactured by docsinnovent (www.docsinnovent.com). The v-gel is available in various sizes, can be positioned quickly, avoids airway trauma, and can be auto-claved for use in multiple patients. However, it is somewhat bulky, making access to the cheek teeth difficult in some patients (Fig. 9.27).

If intubation has been tried unsuccessfully, or if the rabbit is very small, anesthetic maintenance can be accomplished by placing a small anesthetic mask over only the nose, or by using a 4–8 French red rubber catheter inserted into one nostril and advanced to the depth of the pharynx.[13] The catheter is attached to the anesthetic hose using an endotracheal tube adapter (Fig. 9.28).

Heart rate can be monitored via pediatric stethoscope, Doppler blood pressure monitor (crystal can be held or taped directly over the fur of the chest in most patients), or a lingual SpO_2 sensor placed on a foot, ear, or scrotum. Visualization of

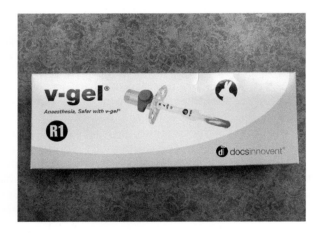

Figure 9.27   The v-gel endotracheal tube.

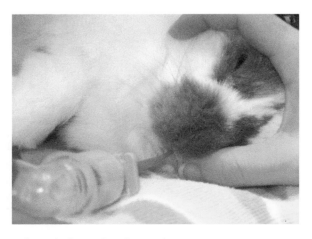

Figure 9.28   Rabbit with nasal tube in place for anesthetic maintenance.

the mucous membrane color (tongue is especially useful) and the chest movements of respirations is essential. The palpebral reflex is lost by rabbits early in light planes of anesthesia, followed by the pedal withdrawal reflex. At a surgical plane, the auricular reflex is lost. If the corneal reflex has been lost, this indicates that the patient is too deep. Rabbits are prone to developing hypothermia, so be sure to monitor and maintain body temperature (see web content: Fig. 9.29W).

Rabbits are very sensitive to pain, becoming anorectic and lethargic. Gastrointestinal (GI) stasis, delayed wound healing, shock, and death can result. Tooth grinding is a common sign of pain in rabbits, as are hunching, vocalization, and inactivity. Any rabbit with a painful condition or who is undergoing a painful procedure should be provided with pain relief. Analgesics useful in rabbits include buprenorphine, butorphanol, meloxicam, and carprofen.

Common Dental Problems of Rabbits

Malocclusion

A common problem in lagomorphs is dental malocclusion, causing tooth overgrowth[6] (see web content: Figs. 9.30W and 9.31W). Malocclusions are classified as traumatic or atraumatic. Traumatic malocclusions result from injury to a tooth causing a loss of a portion of the crown and subsequently the loss of normal wear on the opposing tooth. Atraumatic malocclusions normally result from hereditary conditions such as jaw length disparity or nutritional deficiencies such as not consuming enough roughage to wear down the continually growing teeth. In either case, tooth overgrowth can result in an altered curvature of the teeth so that the occlusal surfaces are no longer able to meet and wear down adequately. Altered curvature of the teeth can also widen the spaces in between teeth, leading to food and debris impaction, periodontal pockets, and periodontal abscesses.

Inadequately worn teeth can lead to sharp spikes, causing soft tissue lacerations of the tongue and buccal mucosa. Excess salivation ("slobbers") can occur. Tooth root elongation can occur secondary to crown elongation, when the elongated crowns come into contact with the opposing teeth and eventually are prevented from further eruption. In this case eruption stops but tooth growth does not, so the root apices begin to intrude into the bone of the mandible and maxilla. Elongation of the mandibular roots can cause bone remodeling and a palpable "lumpy jaw," while long maxillary cheek tooth roots can break into the orbit, causing eye prolapse in severe cases. Root elongation of the maxillary incisors can obstruct the lacrimal ducts, causing lacrimal discharge (see web content: Fig. 9.32W).

Traumatic malocclusions are treated by smoothing the edges of the fractured tooth with a bur or file, treating the pulp, if exposed, by removing any infected tissue with a sterile, small round bur and capping it with calcium hydroxide paste topped with a thin layer of glass ionomer. Routine odontoplasty (also referred to as crown height reduction or occlusal leveling) should also be performed on the opposing tooth until the fractured tooth regrows.[1] Atraumatic malocclusions due to jaw length disparity can be treated, although not usually cured because the underlying jaw malocclusion remains, with routine odontoplasty, usually every 6–8 weeks for the remainder of the animal's life. This is often also the case when malocclusion has occurred secondary to some other cause such as inadequate dietary roughage. If a tooth's curvature has been altered, causing it not to be able to meet its opposing tooth and wear down, it is uncommon for the curvature to return to normal, even after numerous occlusal leveling procedures.

Extraction of the affected teeth along with the opposing teeth is another option to resolve the problem, and dietary changes such as substituting hay for less abrasive pellets can be successful in cases of nutritional deficiencies where tooth curvature has not been altered, although getting rabbits to accept a new food regimen is often difficult.

Odontoplasty

The use of nail clippers or tooth trimmers to trim incisors or cheek teeth is no longer acceptable as these can cause longitudinal tooth fractures.[14] A much better instrument for performing odontoplasty is a dental bur.[11] To trim the incisors, a #330, #701, or coarse diamond cone bur on a high-speed handpiece with the water turned off can be used, sometimes even in the awake patient. Half of a tongue depressor or a couple of cotton-tipped applicators are inserted into the mouth behind the incisors to protect the tongue and soft tissues from injury. One incisor is cut and shaped at a time, taking care not to cut so much as to enter the pulp chamber (if the pulp does become exposed, treat with calcium hydroxide and glass ionomer as described above) (see web content: Fig. 9.33W).

For odontoplasty of the cheek teeth, the patient must be anesthetized. The rabbit is placed in dorsal recumbency with cheek dilators and mouth gag in place to allow access to the caudal oral cavity. Be sure to protect the tongue and oral tissues from laceration as rabbits can rapidly exsanguinate from such injuries. A slow-speed handpiece and bur such as an HP5, HP558, or lab bur is used to shorten any overgrown teeth or tooth aspects (see web content: Fig. 9.34W). Cotton-tipped applicators or a saliva ejector suction tip with the end cut off and a urinary catheter inserted into it can be used to remove debris from the mouth. This is particularly important if the rabbit is not intubated (see web content: Fig. 9.35W).

If no burs are available, the cheek teeth may be "floated" using small mammal premolar and molar rasps.

Extraction

Extraction can be considered for patients whose teeth are causing ongoing problems. The area should first be rinsed with chlorhexidine solution. Because of the long, curved nature of the tooth roots, a rabbit incisor or premolar/molar luxator should be alternately inserted into the mesial and distal aspects of the periodontal ligament space of each tooth and held in place for 10–20 seconds until it becomes loose.[11] Before extracting the tooth, it should be pressed back up into the alveolus while rotating the tooth slightly to remove the germinal tissue at the open root apex. If no plug of tissue is seen at the apex once the tooth is extracted, there is likely still germinal tissue remaining within the alveolus, and it should be curetted to prevent regrowth. If even a tiny amount of germinal tissue is left behind, the tooth may regrow, so owners must be made aware of this possibility. The extraction sites should be sutured closed with a fine, absorbable suture. If a tooth fractures during extraction, it can be capped with calcium hydroxide and allowed to regrow. Another attempt at extraction can be done at a later time. Remember that the opposing tooth will continue to grow. Odontoplasty or extraction of the opposing tooth may be necessary (see web content: Fig. 9.36W).

Periodontal Disease and Tooth Root Abscess

Plaque-related periodontal disease is rare in rabbits.[6] More commonly, debris such as food or bedding becomes impacted between teeth, which introduces bacteria into the periodontium, resulting in attachment loss (see web content: Fig. 9.37W). The infection can travel down the tooth, causing it to loosen and/or develop a periapical abscess. This infection can affect multiple teeth and may even cause osteomyelitis. Other causes of periapical abscess include pulp exposure and subsequent endodontic infection or penetrating wounds. Treatment involves extraction of the affected teeth, curettage of any infected material and flushing the area with saline or povidone-iodine solution, and systemic antibiotics. Placement of a perioceutic gel or antibiotic-impregnated beads into cleaned periodontal pockets or defects may be considered.[6] Extraoral abscess lancing may be necessary when complete curettage of the abscess is unable to be achieved from within the mouth (see web content: Figs. 9.38W–9.40W). Even with treatment, recurrence of rabbit abscesses is very common, possibly due to the difficulty in complete removal of abscess material, and multiple procedures may be required.

Dental Instruments

A complete set of rabbit dental instruments comprises an incisor luxator, molar/premolar luxator, molar/premolar extraction forceps, root elevators, mouth gag, cheek dilators, molar/premolar rasp, tongue depressor, low-speed burs to use for odontoplasty (HP5, HP8, HP558), and high-speed burs for use in incisor trimming (FG330, FG701) (see web content: Fig. 9.41W). Other useful tools include magnifying loupes, a saliva ejector suction tip fitted with a urinary catheter to suction fluid and debris from the mouth, and cotton-tipped applicators to staunch blood flow, absorb fluid, and remove debris from the mouth.

Husbandry and Home Care

Patients who have had oral surgery may need nutritional support until healed. Lagomorphs may be offered or force-fed a variety of soft foods, such as Oxbow Critical Care, yogurt, or pureed food made from hay, vegetables, and water pureed in a blender. A 35 mL syringe with catheter tip works well to force-feed larger rabbits, while abscess-flushing syringes with the tips trimmed off halfway work well for small rabbits.

Distasteful medications may be mixed with apple juice or another fruit juice in the dosing syringe to improve palatability. If the patient has had extraoral surgery, such as abscess lancing, bedding and debris may stick to the site. Owners should be advised to keep the area clean using a cloth and warm water several times daily. A "weak-tea" solution of povidone-iodine and water, or sterile saline can be used to flush abscesses, making sure not to flush with too much liquid, as these abscesses often still communicate into the oral cavity, and the rabbit must be allowed time to swallow the saline.

To aid in preventing dietary-related malocclusions, owners should be encouraged to feed rabbits the majority of their diets as roughage, such as timothy hay, fresh greens, and vegetables; at most, one-third of their diets should consist of commercial pellets.

Ferret Dentistry

Ferrets are obligate carnivores belonging to the Mustelidae family, which includes weasels, mink, and skunks. They are diphyodont, having a set of deciduous teeth that are replaced by permanent teeth by 9 months of age. Their dentition resembles that of the cat and, like cats, their teeth have true anatomical roots and do not continuously grow.

Oral Anatomy and Dentition of Ferrets

$$2(I3/3, C1/1, P3/3, M1/2) = 30$$

Ferrets have long, narrow, flat skulls, with a short facial region.[15] Like cats, they are missing all first premolars.[16] They are also missing the upper second molars and the lower third molars. The upper fourth premolars have three roots (Figs. 9.42, 9.43 and see web content: Chart 9.5W Ferret Dental Assessment Chart).

Oral Examination of Ferrets

Oral examination can usually be done on pet ferrets while awake. The face should first be examined for asymmetry, swellings, and ocular or nasal discharge, and the submandibular lymph nodes palpated. Check for proper occlusion of the jaws and individual teeth, as well as any tooth fractures, wear, and tartar accumulation. The gums and oral mucosa should be checked for redness, swelling, and oral masses.

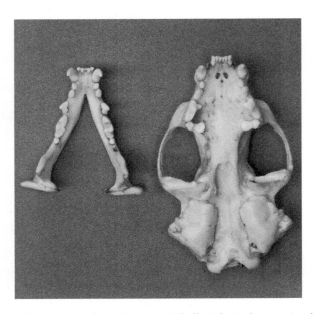

Figure 9.42   Ferret skull: occlusal surfaces (Courtesy of Skulls Unlimited International Inc.).

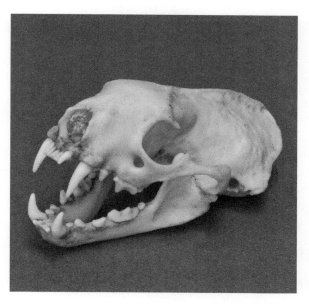

Figure 9.43   Ferret skull: side view (Courtesy of Skulls Unlimited International Inc.).

Table 9.3   Common drug dosages for ferret dentistry

Use	Agent	Dosage
Premedication	Acepromazine	0.1–0.2 mg/kg SC, IM
	Dexmedetomidine	0.04–0.1 mg/kg IM
	Glycopyrrolate	0.01–0.02 mg/kg SC, IM, IV
Anesthesia	Propofol	3–6 mg/kg IV
	Ketamine/diazepam	10–25 mg/kg (K)/1–5 mg/kg (D) IV
Analgesia	Meloxicam	0.1–0.3 mg/kg SC, PO
	Buprenorphine	0.01–0.03 mg/kg IM, SC, IV

IM, intramuscular; SC, subcutaneous; IV, intravenous; PO, per os.
Source: Adapted from Hawkins and Pascoe.[13]

Anesthesia and Pain Management

Preanesthetic fasting should be limited to 2 hours as ferrets are prone to hypoglycemia.[17] A full physical examination and a blood profile consisting of, at minimum, a PCV and total protein should be performed prior to anesthesia, either on the same day as the procedure or on the days leading up to it.[13] Blood collection is facilitated by using a 25 gauge needle on a 1–3 mL syringe from the jugular, cephalic, or lateral saphenous veins. Premedication drugs such as acepromazine, oxymorphone or hydromorphone, and glycopyrrolate are commonly used to provide sedation, supply pain relief, and decrease salivary secretions. An intravenous catheter can be placed in the cephalic or saphenous vein, and intravenous induction can be accomplished with ketamine and diazepam, or propofol[13] (Table 9.3). The ferret's jaw is often tight even once anesthetic induction is

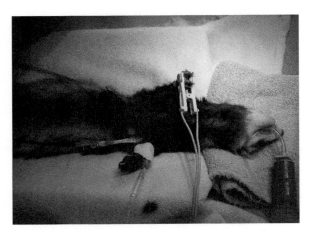

Figure 9.44   Ferret under general anesthesia for routine dental prophylaxis.

complete, but even so, intubation is generally not much more difficult than intubation of the cat. A laryngoscope with a pediatric blade is used to visualize the entrance to the trachea, and a few drops of 2% lidocaine are applied to the arytenoid cartilages before intubation with a 3.0 mm endotracheal tube.[17] Lidocaine gel can also be applied to the end of the endotracheal tube in place of nonmedicated gel lubricant. Isoflurane or sevoflurane provide excellent general anesthesia once the patient is intubated.

Anesthetic monitoring can be performed as for the cat: SpO_2, CO_2, ECG, Doppler or noninvasive blood pressure, temperature, respiration rate, mucous membrane color, and so on can all be easily assessed. Maintenance of body temperature is of particular concern as ferrets are susceptible to hypothermia (Fig. 9.44).

Pain management includes any opioids used in premedication, intraoperative injectables such as meloxicam, buprenorphine, or constant rate infusions (CRIs) of drugs such as ketamine and fentanyl, as well as dental regional nerve blocks using lidocaine or bupivicaine.[4] The infraorbital, mental, mandibular, and maxillary blocks can be performed on the ferret in much the same manner as in the cat, with the maximum dose of local anesthetic being 2 mg/kg. Postoperatively, oral liquid pain medications such as meloxicam can be administered at home by the owner.

Common Dental Problems of Ferrets

Periodontal Disease

Ferret periodontal disease is staged and treated in the same manner as is periodontal disease in dogs and cats.[17] Mild tartar accumulation AND gingivitis warrants a complete professional dental prophylaxis under general anesthesia (Fig. 9.45). Moderate to severe periodontal disease will require not only a complete prophylaxis but also intraoral dental radiographs to assess the degree of attachment loss (see web content: Figs. 9.46W and 9.47W). Periodontal therapy such as subgingival curettage and root planing, or tooth extraction can then be performed. Periodontal therapy and extraction are accomplished in the same manner as in the dog and cat, with extraction sites being sutured closed, and using appropriate antibiotic therapy and pain management.

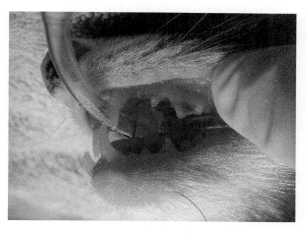

Figure 9.45   Ferret with tartar accumulation and mild gingivitis.

Tooth Fracture

Tooth fracture, especially of the canine teeth, is very common in the ferret due to their tendency to chew on many household surfaces, including cage bars, chair legs, and children's toys[16] (see web content: Fig. 9.48W). If a fracture has exposed the tooth pulp, treatment is necessary to prevent or eliminate infection. If the pulp is not exposed, radiographs should still be obtained to ensure that the trauma that caused the fracture did not also cause pulp death. The root of the canine tooth in the ferret is longer than its crown, a factor that can make extraction of a fractured but otherwise periodontally healthy canine tooth difficult. Root canal therapy can be performed in these teeth just as it is done in a canine tooth of a cat, and has the advantage of allowing the ferret to maintain a functional dentition while minimizing recovery time and postsurgical pain (see web content: Fig. 9.49W).

Dental Instruments

The periodontal probes, explorers, dental mirrors, scalers, and curettes used for feline prophylaxis function well in the ferret's mouth. The same applies to dental surgical instruments: Feline periosteal elevators, luxators, extraction forceps, root tip picks, needle drivers, forceps, and small scalpel blades such as #15 are sufficient to make up a ferret oral surgery tray. Dental suction units or gauze packing can be used to keep fluids and debris from entering the trachea during procedures.

Husbandry and Home Care

Ferrets are carnivorous, requiring high-protein diets from animal sources to obtain essential amino acids;[17] 20–30% of their diet should come from fat. There are many commercial diets for ferrets. Ensure that the ones your clients are feeding meet the above guidelines. Small amounts of fruits, vegetables, and grains can be offered, although refined carbohydrates should be avoided. Tartar accumulation and perio-dontal disease seem to develop in ferrets regardless if they are fed a dry or a moist diet.[18]

If a ferret has developed anorexia due to dental disease or postoperatively, syringe-feeding a canned high-protein diet such as Hill's a/d (Hill's Pet Nutrition Inc., Topeka, KS) should be performed until the ferret will eat on its own. Most ferrets will tolerate feedings of 8–12 mL three to four times daily.[19] Medications should be dispensed in liquid form if possible, as it can be very difficult for ferret owners to successfully administer pills or capsules.

To prevent the development of periodontal disease, ferrets can be taught to accept daily toothbrushing. Use a cat-sized toothbrush and pet toothpaste.

Dental Radiography for the Exotic Patient

Materials and Equipment

Dental radiography for the exotic patient is best performed with a conventional dental X-ray unit. Good-quality radiographs can be obtained using either manual or digital systems. If a dental X-ray unit is unavailable, a standard X-ray unit capable of producing 45–70 kilovoltage (kVp) and 300 milliamperes (mA) in 0.008–0.016 seconds[20] can be used to obtain extraoral radiographs of larger rodents and rabbits; however, the correct positioning for each view is more difficult to achieve, and the fine resolution of nonscreen dental X-ray films provide much better detail than standard films in cassettes.[1] Sedation or general anesthesia is required to ensure that the patient does not move during exposure; most of these patients are small enough that attempting to restrain their heads "by hand" while wearing bulky leaded gloves usually does not prevent them from squirming and can also obscure areas of interest on the resulting radiograph.

Rodents and Rabbits

Skull radiographs are a necessary part of the complete oral examination in rabbits and rodents as they allow assessment of crown and root length, the occlusal plane, any periapical lucencies, or other bony changes. Extraoral skull radiographs are pre-ferred for these species as the small size of their oral cavities makes it difficult even to insert film, much less obtain a diagnostic image. Manual dental film size 4 will capture the entire skull of most species, or several exposures taken with a size 2 digi-tal dental sensor can be compiled together to get a complete picture of the maxilla and mandible.

There are four skull views that should be obtained in order to properly diagnose pathology: lateral, two lateral obliques, and dorsoventral.[21] The lateral view is the most useful, allowing assessment of the patient's occlusion, crown or root over-growth, and any bony changes to the ventral mandible.[16] The drawback to this view is that the left and right quadrants of the mouth are superimposed (Figs. 9.50 and 9.51). The two lateral obliques, which are taken at approximately 45 degrees

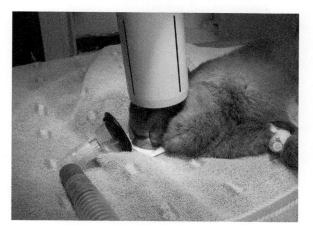

Figure 9.50   Lateral dental radiograph positioning on a rabbit.

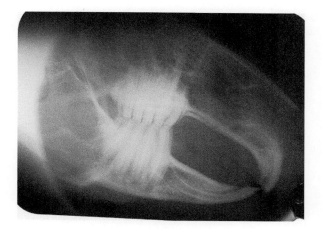

Figure 9.51   Lateral dental radiograph of a rabbit with normal occlusion.

right-to-left and left-to-right, show details of individual root apices and their surrounding bone without superimposition of structures on the opposite side of the mouth (Figs. 9.52 and 9.53). The dorsoventral view shows the symmetry (or asymmetry) of the skull, and any irregularity to the contours of the bone including that of the orbits (Fig. 9.54).

An additional view that is of particular use in guinea pigs is the rostrocaudal view, where the patient is placed in dorsal recumbency, nose pointing up at the X-ray tube head, and the film placed beneath the skull. Due to the occlusal angulation of the cheek teeth in guinea pigs, this view is the best to visualize whether occlusal abnormalities are present; normal guinea pig occlusion will result in an oblique radiolucent line between the upper and lower cheek teeth on either side of the mouth[22] (see web content: Fig. 9.55W). All radiographs should be assessed for the following: elongation of the roots (see web content: Figs. 9.56W and 9.57W); the shape of occlusal surfaces – normal incisors are chisel-shaped and cheek teeth have an even "zigzag" pattern, whereas waves or steps are signs of malocclusion (see web content: Fig. 9.58W); and a fine radiolucent line should exist between the alveolar bone and

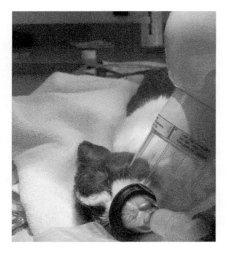

Figure 9.52   Lateral oblique radiograph positioning on a rabbit.

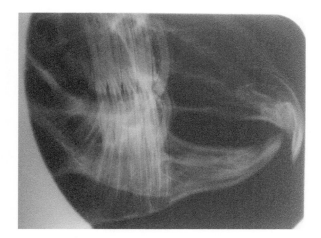

Figure 9.53   Lateral oblique radiograph of a rabbit.

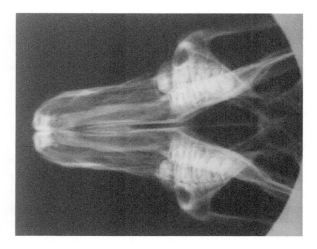

Figure 9.54   Dorsoventral radiograph of a rabbit.

the subgingival crown, while absence of this can indicate ankylosis, and areas of increased bone lucency may indicate abscessation.[23]

Ferrets

Ferret dental radiographs are obtained for the same reasons as dental radiographs are obtained in dogs and cats: to determine the degree of attachment loss in cases of periodontal disease, pulp exposure and periapical changes in cases of tooth fracture, assessment of oral masses, and evaluation of many other oral problems including missing or impacted teeth, retained roots, nonvital teeth, jaw fractures, and so on.

Positioning for dental radiography is much the same as that for the cat. Extraoral skull radiographs are not recommended, as small-sized manual dental films (size 0, 1, 2) can be used intraorally to obtain much better quality images without superimposition of oral structures. Bisecting angle technique is used to obtain intraoral images of the maxillary teeth, while parallel technique can be used in most cases to obtain intraoral images of the mandibular premolars and molars.[17] Some digital dental X-ray sensors are too wide to fit within the mouth for standard intraoral views. In this case extraoral oblique views can be taken of the maxillary teeth, while bisecting angle technique can be used to obtain an intraoral view of the mandibular teeth with the X-ray sensor placed perpendicular to the teeth and as far back in the mouth as possible. Intraoral radiographs of the canine teeth can easily be obtained with either manual dental films or digital sensors (see web content: Figs. 9.59W–9.61W).

Further information for veterinary technicians about exotic pet dentistry is provided in Video 9.1 Pocket pet dentistry for the veterinary technician.

References

1. Legendre, L. 2003. Oral disorders of exotic rodents. *Veterinary Clinics of North America Exotic Animal Practice* 6:601–628.
2. Legendre, L. 2016. Anatomy and disorders of the oral cavity of guinea pigs. *Veterinary Clinics: Exotic Animal Practice* 19:825–842.
3. Quesenberry, KE, Donnelly, TM, Hillyer, EV. 2012. Biology, husbandry, and clinical techniques of guinea pigs and chinchillas. In *Ferrets, Rabbits, and Rodents: Clinical Medicine and Surgery*, 3rd edn (ed. KE Quesenberry, JW Carpenter). St. Louis, MO: Saunders, pp. 279–294.
4. Capello, V, Lennox, AM. 2012. Small mammal dentistry. In *Ferrets, Rabbits, and Rodents: Clinical Medicine and Surgery*, 3rd edn (ed. KE Quesenberry), JW Carpenter). St. Louis, MO: Saunders, pp. 452–471.
5. Bennett, RA. 2012. Soft tissue surgery. In *Ferrets, Rabbits, and Rodents: Clinical Medicine and Surgery*, 3rd edn (ed. KE Quesenberry, JW Carpenter. St. Louis, MO: Saunders, pp. 373–391.
6. Berg, ML. 2011. Exotic animal dentistry (CVC in Kansas City Proceedings) http://veterinarycalendar.dvm360.com/exotic-animal-dentistry-proceedings?id=&pageID=1&sk=&date= (accessed January 8, 2018).

CHAPTER 9

7. Lennox, AM, Bauck, L. 2012. Basic anatomy, physiology, husbandry, and clinical techniques. In *Ferrets, Rabbits, and Rodents: Clinical Medicine and Surgery*, 3rd edn (ed. KE Quesenberry, JW Carpenter). St. Louis, MO: Saunders, pp. 339–353.

8. Morrisey, JK, Carpenter, JW. 2012. Formulary. In *Ferrets, Rabbits, and Rodents: Clinical Medicine and Surgery*, 3rd edn (ed. KE Quesenberry, JW Carpenter). St. Louis, MO: Saunders, pp. 566–575.

9. Ivey, E, Carpenter, JW. 2012. African hedgehogs. In *Ferrets, Rabbits, and Rodents: Clinical Medicine and Surgery*, 3rd edn (ed. KE Quesenberry, JW Carpenter). St. Louis, MO: Saunders, pp. 411–427.

10. Ness, RD, Johnson-Delaney, CA. 2012. Sugar gliders. In *Ferrets, Rabbits, and Rodents: Clinical Medicine and Surgery*, 3rd edn (ed. KE Quesenberry, JW Carpenter). St. Louis, MO: Saunders, pp. 393–410.

11. Crossley, DA. 2003. Oral biology and disorders of lagomorphs. *Veterinary Clinics of North America Exotic Animal Practice* 6:629–659.

12. Steinmetz, HW. Dental diseases in rabbits and guinea pigs. In World Small Animal Association World Congress Proceedings, 2010.

13. Hawkins, MG, Pascoe, PJ. 2012. Anesthesia, analgesia, and sedation of small mammals. In *Ferrets, Rabbits, and Rodents: Clinical Medicine and Surgery*, 3rd edn (ed. KE Quesenberry, JW Carpenter). St. Louis, MO: Saunders, pp. 429–451.

14. Lennox, A. 2008. Diagnosis and treatment of dental disease in pet rabbits. *Journal of Exotic Pet Medicine* 17:107–113.

15. Mohamed, R. Anatomical and radiographic study on the skull of the common opossum. *Veterinary Sciences* April 2018.

16. Capello, V, Lennox, AM. 2012. Small mammal dentistry. In *Ferrets, Rabbits, and Rodents: Clinical Medicine and Surgery*, 3rd edn (ed. KE Quesenberry, JW Carpenter). St. Louis, MO: Saunders, pp. 452–471.

17. Cooper, J. 2017. Ferret dentistry: no weasling about it. *Today's Veterinary Nurse* 2(1) https://todaysveterinarynurse.com/articles/ferret-dentistry-no-weaseling-about-it/ (accessed January 8, 2018).

18. Hoefer, HL, Fox, JG, Bell, JA. 2012. Gastrointestinal diseases. In *Ferrets, Rabbits, and Rodents: Clinical Medicine and Surgery*, 3rd edn (ed. KE Quesenberry, JW Carpenter). St. Louis, MO: Saunders, pp. 25–40.

19. Quesenberry, KE, Orcutt, C. 2012. Basic approach to veterinary care. In *Ferrets, Rabbits, and Rodents: Clinical Medicine and Surgery*, 3rd edn (ed. KE Quesenberry, JW Carpenter). St. Louis, MO: Saunders, pp. 13–24.

20. Fischetti, AJ. 2012. Diagnostic imaging. In *Ferrets, Rabbits, and Rodents: Clinical Medicine and Surgery*, 3rd edn (ed. KE Quesenberry, JW Carpenter). St. Louis, MO: Saunders, pp. 502–510.

21. Hoefer, HL. 2000. Small mammal dentistry. In Proceedings: Colorado State Veterinary Medical Association Convention 2000.

22. Capello, V. 2003. Dental diseases and surgical treatment in pet rodents. *Exotic DVM* 5:21–27.

23. Meredith, A. 2007. Rabbit dentistry. *European Journal of Companion Animal Practice* 17(1):55–62.

Discharging the Dental Patient

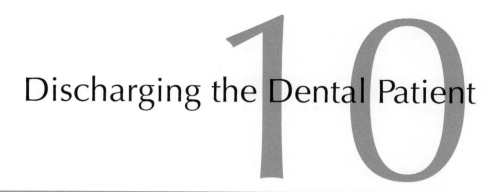

Patricia Dominguez, LVT, VTS (Dentistry)

Learning Objectives

- Effectively communicate with owners about their pet's dental procedures
- Properly demonstrate the importance and value of a high-quality dental program
- Teach owner's how to successfully treat and maintain their pet's oral health.

Small Animal Dental Procedures for Veterinary Technicians and Nurses, Second Edition.
Edited by Jeanne R. Perrone.
© 2021 John Wiley & Sons, Inc. Published 2021 by John Wiley & Sons, Inc.

CHAPTER 10

A complete dental procedure is not finished once the patient is awake from anesthesia. A vital part of veterinary dentistry is to teach the owners how to maintain their pet's oral care at home. They need to understand how important a healthy mouth is to having a healthy body. We have already seen in human medicine how periodontal disease is linked to heart disease, diabetes, low birth weights and even pneumonia.[1] In veterinary medicine we are only beginning to uncover the links between dental disease and overall systemic health problems in our canine and feline companions.[2] It is our responsibility to convey this message at each and every visit, starting with the first puppy and kitten exam. Good communication is essential when explaining to owners about the details of their pet's dental procedure, both at regular exams and as part of a discharge after a dental procedure. Digital pictures, radiographs, models, and charts should be used as tools to illustrate the importance of what was done to their pet. Clients will need to learn the value of every step performed during a dental prophylaxis. This will demonstrate the similarities between the owner's dental check-ups and their pet's dental procedure day.

In this chapter you will learn how to present the value of a high-quality dental procedure. When owners understand the complexity of what is involved, they can then appreciate the value of the services that have been provided. Visual aids are key to ensuring the client appreciates each step of a thorough dental procedure. This establishes the hospital as a trustworthy facility that provides a higher standard of care. Also, cost tends to be less of an issue if they understand the need for any of the treatments provided. Clients will not only continue to return for these services, but will also refer people to you once they are aware of the dangers of periodontal disease.

Proper client education and encouragement is necessary to promote preventative dentistry. Owners need to feel that the complete care of their pet is a team effort and works best when they are involved. Recheck visits and follow-up calls are great opportunities to touch base with clients and review how they are managing oral care at home. If they have started a prescription dental diet, these phone calls can be utilized to remind them of food refills. This will not only increase revenue for the practice, but also help keep pets on the road to better oral health.

Client compliance is crucial to fighting the battle against plaque and tartar accumulation. Once we have cleaned the oral cavity, it is our duty to give owners the tools necessary to be able to provide good oral care at home. If the client understands that the dental procedure is just a part of a complete dental health program, they will be more likely to comply with your recommendations.

Discharge Instructions: What You Need

The Dental Prophylaxis

A dental prophylaxis is described as the cleaning of an oral cavity without periodontal disease or mild gingivitis. The idea is to prevent periodontitis.[3] The discharge instructions for a dental prophylaxis are going to be less involved than the discharge instructions of a pet that had a dental procedure to clean and treat advanced stages of periodontal disease. We will discuss the dental prophylaxis discharge first.

Once the dental cleaning is complete, it is time to organize all of the information necessary for the owners to take home with them. This should include: a complete write-up of everything that was done during their pet's procedure, special instructions regarding home care, and an oral care plan formulated for that particular pet and family to be followed at home. Using these three guidelines will give clients a comprehensive package to understanding their pets oral care needs immediately after a dental procedure and for routine maintenance.

The discharge write-up should contain an explanation of what is entailed in a complete dental prophylaxis. This will educate clients on the numerous steps involved in the cleaning procedure and assure them that their pet received the highest quality in oral care that can be provided. You can use this area to explain the use of injectable antibiotics, pain medications, intravenous fluids, and anesthetic monitoring. Although the use of injectable antibiotics and pain medications is not required for a dental prophylaxis, the practitioner may choose to prescribe them on a case-by-case basis. All of this information can be formulated into a generalized template on any word processing system or hospital management software (see Appendix 7). Once the document has been saved as a template, it is very easy to personalize them for each patient by inserting their name. The report should also include an area where you can insert what was found on oral exam and a description of any treatments performed. This will allow you to tailor each discharge packet based on the pet's procedure.

A vital part of the packet will be the visual aspect. Digital pictures and radiographs make it easy for the client to see the need for and end results of the treatments performed. The packet gives them something tangible to show family members, co-workers and friends who may not be able to understand everything that was done without seeing it for themselves (see Appendices 8 and 9).

The Dental Procedure

A dental procedure involves not only the cleaning of the oral cavity but also the treatment of other dental diseases. Specific instructions will need to be given in the cases of extractions, oral surgery, periodontal, endodontic, or orthodontic therapies. You will also need to outline what the owners should expect after their pet goes home from anesthesia and how to determine if the pet is not doing well after their procedure. This section should also instruct the owner of any medications, special feeding or chewing instructions, and when to return for a recheck. Be sure to include contact information for the dental team involved with their pet's procedure in case they have any questions or concerns.

Examining the pet after extractions or when advanced dental therapies are performed gives you the opportunity to evaluate the oral cavity and gingival healing. The owner will be able to describe any differences in the pet's chewing behavior and personality. Use this time to reiterate the importance of home care and make a timeline to check their progress before their oral condition worsens again.

The most significant component of the dental discharge process is formulating an oral care regimen that can be incorporated into the pet's daily routine. Emphasis needs to be put on the value of home care in minimizing the accumulation of bacteria and plaque in the mouth. You will need to assess the pet's personality and the commitment level of the family to preventing dental disease. Use this opportunity to explain how to introduce their pet to having their teeth brushed. The owners will also need ways of remembering to brush their pet's teeth on a daily basis. This can be as simple as putting the toothbrush and toothpaste next to their own in the bathroom so when they brush their teeth, they know it is time to brush their pet's teeth as well. To get more tips, review the lessons learned on home care in Chapter 5.

The Dental Discharge Experience

Many clients will have experienced being discharged in a noisy waiting room where they are given their pet and a sheet of instructions. This will need to change if you want to ensure your clients have a good comprehension of what was done to their pet and have all of their questions answered. This can only be done if you take the time to go over all of the details of their pet's dental procedure and home instructions.

When discharging a patient after a dental procedure, you want to make sure you have a quiet area where there are no distractions. It is a good idea to have a room set aside where you can utilize educational tools such as models, skulls, diagrams, books, and albums (Fig. 10.1). It works well to have a photo album prepared to show clients with pictures of common dental issues, treatment options, and advanced dental procedures. It is easier for owners to understand the importance of dental radiographs when they can see examples of tooth resorption, tooth root infections, oral masses, impacted teeth, and persistent deciduous teeth. This album can be used to educate clients both before and after a dental procedure. I have found that keeping digital folders on computers throughout the hospital or on a communal tablet is very effective in demonstrating dental pathology. It is also helpful to have a view box or a monitor where dental radiographs and digital pictures can be viewed (Figs. 10.2 and 10.3). Utilize technology to record and show videos that promote your staff and demonstrate to proper way to brush pet's teeth or apply oral gels and rinses.

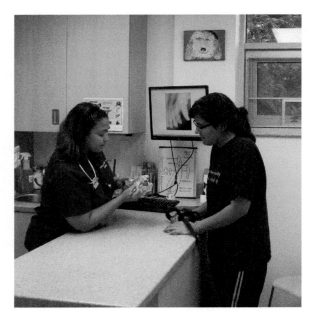

Figure 10.1　Technician explaining the dental procedure using a skull and a periodontal probe (Courtesy of Gotham Veterinary Center).

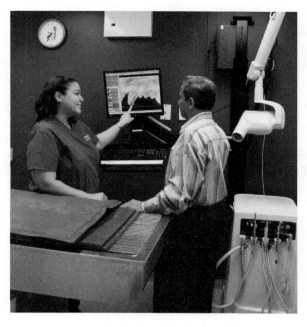

Figure 10.2   Technician showing a dental radiograph to the owner. This gives a visual component to add to the explanation of the dental procedure (Courtesy of Gotham Veterinary Center).

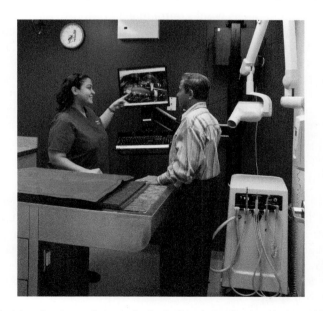

Figure 10.3   Technician showing a photograph of a finding during the dental exam. This gives a visual component that contributes to the explanation of the procedure (Courtesy of Gotham Veterinary Center).

This discharge room is also a great place to have samples of toothbrushes, toothpaste, oral gels, rinses, water additives, dental diets, and dental chews. Instruct the family on the benefits and use of each product before deciding on a daily care regimen that will work for them. Since all of this can be overwhelming to an owner, be sure to have handouts available they can review later. To minimize paper use, you can opt to email the instructional aids to clients or have links reviewing oral care on the hospital's website or on social media. But remember, nothing is as effective as showing an owner how to brush their pet's teeth so they can see how easily it can be accomplished.

Once you have gone over the entire dental procedure with the client using pictures, given special instructions, discussed medications, home care, answered all questions, and addressed all concerns, only then should you reunite them with their pet. If you introduce the pet at the beginning, their attention will usually be more focused on the pet than on what you are saying. Try to present the pet looking as close as possible to what it looked like when the owner left it in your care. Dental procedures will involve large amounts of moisture around the pet's face so take a few minutes while the pet is recovering to clean, dry, and brush the hair around it.

A follow-up call should be made to the owners to check on the status of the pet after the dental procedure. This will allow you to address any problems before they return for their recheck visit.

Advanced Dental Procedure Release

An advanced dental procedure may involve major oral surgery. These procedures are extensive and will require a more involved recovery. Patients will need to be on a softened food diet, restricted activity, and will need to take daily medications. Owners should be told and shown exactly which teeth were removed or repaired. This will help them avoid certain areas while continuing an oral care regimen at home.

Oral sutures will need to be left intact for proper healing of the gingival tissue.

It is advisable to list any abnormal signs to look for that would be a cause for concern. If your facility is not accessible 24 hours a day, you should include contact information for either a doctor on call or a local emergency clinic in case they need assistance throughout the night. These are major procedures and pet owners need to have guidance in what to look for during the first few days of recovery and who to call if they have questions or concerns.

The Importance of Photographs and Radiographs

Sometimes we have to put ourselves in the shoes of our clients to understand what they are seeing and feeling. Imagine for a moment you take your car to an auto care center. You might get a phone call during the day explaining the work needed and you give your consent for them to proceed. When you go to pick up your car, you are handed a bill for almost $1000.00 and your keys. Would you appreciate the real value of what you spent?

Value is often measured by the way it is perceived. The field of veterinary medicine is based on client relationships and patient care. Pet parents want to know that they can trust you with members of their family and that you will do what is in the pet's best interest. One way to build this bond is by taking the time and effort to create informational discharge packets which show what was done to the pet during the course of the day (Fig. 10.4). I have even incorporated ways of engaging pet owners while their pet is with us. In today's world, a simple text or picture can help calm the nerves of any anxious pet owner (see web content: Fig. 10.5W). We take a picture of the pet in the arms of

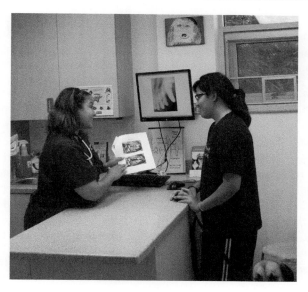

Figure 10.4 Technician going over the discharge packet with the owner (Courtesy of Gotham Veterinary Center).

one of our caring staff members and send it to the owner before the procedure with an update of how their day is going. Pet parents really appreciate the updates and love the pictures. Within minutes, you can see these pictures posted on social media with a tag back to your clinic. This is another easy, cost-free way to promote your practice and at the same time make your clients very happy.

Dentistry is a topic that is better understood when it is seen instead of being heard. The perception of value will increase when the client is presented with before and after pictures. This can be accomplished by using a digital camera or cell phone able to take high-resolution pictures of objects at a very close distance. The digital pictures can be exported into a template that will demonstrate the difference of each side before and after the dental procedure. Be sure to include close ups of any problem areas and copies of any radiographs taken. These visual aids will show the owner exactly what was done and the reasons why it was necessary.

Pictures really are worth a thousand words. They are clear indications of abnormal findings and show drastic changes after the treatment plan has been implemented. A copy of the pictures and dental radiographs should be saved in the patient's medical record to refer back to during future dental procedures. Sending home a copy with the owners or emailing them a digital version will serve as a reminder of signs to look for in their pet's mouth. It can also serve as a motivational tool to adhere to a daily oral care regimen.

Dental radiography has become a necessary standard when providing a high level of oral care. It is impossible to perform a complete dental assessment without incorporating a complete set of dental radiographs. Research has shown that the majority of pathology will be found underneath the gumline. The American Animal Hospital Association (AAHA) guidelines specify that all pets should receive a full set of dental radiographs to establish a baseline evaluation of a pet's oral health, in addition to taking specific radiographs when abnormal findings are discovered on oral exam.[4]

Dental radiology plays a vital role in assessing any abnormalities found during the oral exam. Dental radiographs are also needed when performing procedures that will alter the pet's oral cavity. You will need radiographs before any treatment to justify its recommendation. After extractions are done radiographs can confirm that all tooth root material was removed and that no damage was done to the surrounding teeth or bone.

Whether you are developing dental radiographs or have a digital unit, clients will love seeing the details of their pet's dental treatment. If you are developing radiographs you can take digital pictures of them on a view box or use a radiograph scanner to convert them to digital pictures. If you are using a digital dental radiography unit, it is easy to export the images into a document template. Any photo editing software will allow you to attach text notes to the pictures. Utilize this feature to illustrate what pathology was discovered in the oral cavity and on the dental radiographs. Clients will often put these pictures in a place at their home or workplace where others will see them. In today's world, we will typically see these pictures posted on social media which allows for others to become educated about the type of dental work done at your practice. This is a great tool to promote your practice's dental program. You can personalize the discharge packet and pictures by adding your hospital's name, contact information, and logo. This will lead people to associate your clinic with providing a higher level of dental care.

Managing Recheck Visits

Recheck visits are a great opportunity to connect with clients and reevaluate the pet's oral cavity. Clients should be instructed to return for a follow-up after any extractions or oral surgery. At this visit you should make sure the gum tissue is healing properly and that the pet is doing well at home. This is also the best time to reiterate the importance of home care. Owners of pets receiving true dental prophylaxis (just cleanings) will also benefit from follow-up visits. After paying a large bill, most people want to know how to avoid another extensive dental procedure. The answer is to brush, brush, brush! (Fig. 10.6). When you sit down with the family to discuss the discharge instructions, a home care regimen will need to be formulated and then implemented. Your goal should be to teach them that brushing is the most beneficial to their pet's oral health care. If daily brushing is not possible then introduce them to the alternatives such as oral gels, rinses, dental diets, and dental chews. These can be incorporated into a multimodal approach to keep their pet's oral cavity free from bacteria. Show the family how the program you design for them will help prevent the accumulation of plaque and thus the formation of tartar. All of these daily treatments are to reduce the effects of periodontal disease and extend the time needed between professional cleanings. Well-trained staff members are crucial to educating clients on the use of all the oral care products available. Having a point person responsible for oral health education will give clients a person to contact when they need help or have questions.

Most veterinary scheduling software used today will allow you to pull reports on recent dental procedures or clients who have purchased oral care products, dental diets, or dental chews. You should also be able to incorporate a call back system in the software where it will remind you to call clients a few days, a few months, and a year after a dental procedure. This will allow you to monitor the success of the oral care regimen discussed at the discharge appointment. If the owner is having a difficult time with compliance, try to reevaluate the home care program and adjust it to fit their needs. Offer to have the owner come in to discuss tips and tricks to make the process go smoother. Often, the hardest part of the process is getting the owner

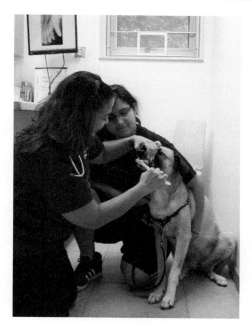

Figure 10.6 Technician demonstrating toothbrushing (Courtesy of Gotham Veterinary Center).

to remember to take on this initiative every day. Advise them to put the oral care products in a place they will see every day, like next to their own toothbrush, next to the pet's food, or next to the pet's leash. These daily reminders should help encourage them to take a few minutes out of each day to help their pet on the road to better oral health. If the owner is doing a good job with complying, then continue giving them support and guidance to continue. Positive reinforcement will make the goal of good oral care at home more attainable.

Reminders: How Often Should Dental Patients Return?

Pets should have their teeth evaluated every 6–12 months. The need for a cleaning will depend on how often the owners are able to provide oral care at home, what the pet is chewing on, and genetics. The more compliant an owner is with daily brushing the less need there will be for another anesthetic procedure to professionally clean the teeth. Prevention is a big part of fighting dental disease. The recheck visit should not only emphasize monitoring home care but also be the opportunity to identify problems before they become serious.

Offering free or low-cost dental evaluations will encourage clients to bring their pets more frequently instead of waiting until it is too late. Use this time to show the owner how prevention is more cost effective than performing major dental treatment plans. Routine maintenance prophylaxis not only is less expensive, but is also less traumatic and requires less anesthesia than more extensive dental procedures. This should make your clients feel more comfortable and understanding of the benefits of preventative dentistry.

Since bacteria start to reattach to the enamel within hours of a dental cleaning, it is imperative to begin an oral care routine as soon as possible. Just like with us, the more you brush and floss, the cleaner your teeth will be. The same theory applies to our pets in that a healthy mouth is a healthy body. By keeping their mouths clean we can help them live healthier, longer lives.

As a health care team, you should construct a plan for follow-up visits with every patient undergoing any dental treatments. The patients that are prone to periodontal disease should be seen more frequently. By seeing them every few months you have the opportunity to intervene when you see the signs of early periodontal disease. Patients that are less prone to periodontal disease can be seen every 6 months to ensure proper home care cleaning techniques are being followed.

Each recheck visit should include a review of how the pet is doing at home, including eating and chewing behaviors. You should discuss any problems that may have come up trying to provide oral care at home. It is also a good opportunity to share information about new dental procedures and products with clients. By starting these relationships, you will build everlasting bonds that will help our patients live longer, healthier lives by staying on the road to good oral health.

References

1. DeBowes, LJ. 1998. The effects of dental disease on systemic disease. *Veterinary Clinics of North America Small Animal Practice* 28:1057–1062.
2. DeBowes, LJ, Mosier, D, Logan, E et al. 1996. Association of periodontal disease and histologic lesions in multiple organs from 45 dogs. *Journal of Veterinary Dentistry* 13:57–60.
3. Holmstrom, SE. 2000. *Veterinary Dentistry for the Technician and Office Staff.* Philadelphia: WB Saunders.
4. Bellows, J, Berg, ML, Dennis S et al. 2019. *AAHA Dental Care Guidelines for Dogs and Cats.* https://www.aaha.org/globalassets/02-guidelines/dental/aaha_dental_guidelines.pdf (accessed March 2020).

Appendices

Appendix 1   Home Oral Health Care Interview Form

(To help formulate a plan for successful home care.)

Relationship with the Pet

- Is your pet a:
  - (a) Family member   ☐
  - (b) Outdoor pet   ☐
  - (c) Guard dog   ☐
  - (d) Working dog   ☐
- What is the dental problem? (Check all that apply)
  - (a) Bad breath   ☐
  - (b) Mobile teeth   ☐
  - (c) Missing teeth   ☐
  - (d) Heavy tartar accumulation   ☐
  - (e) Trouble eating   ☐
  - (f) Difficulty when chewing   ☐
- Are there financial concerns that would impact your choice of products? Yes ☐ or No ☐
- Are you able to provide oral home care? Yes ☐ or No ☐
- Are there any medical considerations that limit your ability to provide home care? Yes ☐ or No ☐

Patient Information

- Is your pet likely to cooperate with home care? Yes ☐ or No ☐
- Would your pet cooperate with daily toothbrushing? Yes ☐ or No ☐
- Does your pet have any medical or anatomical considerations that make one form of treatment preferable to another? Yes ☐ or No ☐

APPENDICES

Environment

- What is your pet's current diet?_____
- What treats does your pet get on a regular basis?_____
- What toys does your pet chew on or play with on a regular basis? _____
_____

- Does your pet destroy toys within 5–10 minutes? _____
_____

- Are there other pets in the household? _____
- Do you have time in your day to perform daily brushing? _____
_____

Our Recommendations _____

Courtesy of Judy Ozier, CVT, VTS (Dentistry)

Appendix 2   Canine Dental Chart

Clinic name: _____

Doctor name: _____   Phone: _____

Date: _____   Fax: _____

Client name: _____   Client #: _____

Patient name: _____   Age ____ Sex: ____ Breed: _____

Color: _____ Weight: _____ Allergies: _____

Medical alert			
Chief complaint			
Past dental history			
Pertinent history			
Diet			
Home care	Brush	Rinse	Medications
Other			

Initial Exam		
SKULL TYPE	**DENTAL ABNORMALITIES**	**MISC**
Brachycephalic	Ret. deciduous _____	Oral enlargements
Mesocephalic	Missing _____	
Dolichocephalic	Supernumerary _____	Pharynx
Other	Caries _____	TMJ
OCCLUSION	Broken _____	
Normal scissors	Discolored _____	Other
Class I:	Gingival recession _____	
PM shift		
Anterior crossbite	**INDEXES**	
Posterior crossbite	Overall calculus index (CI)	
Rostrally deviated max K9	(0) None	
Base narrow lower canines	(I) Supragingival/w sl. subgingival	
Class II:	(II) Moderate subgingival	
Brachygnathic/over	(III) Abundant supragingival and/or subgingival	
Class III (prognathic/under):	Gingivitis index (GI)	
Level/ reverse scissor/	(0) None	
underbite	(I) Mild/no bleeding	
Other:	(II) Moderate/bleeding on probing	
Wry	(III) Severe/spontaneous bleeding	
Occlusal wear		
ICPM		

Physical Exam				
Temperature:	F	Pulse (bpm):		Respiratory rate:
CRT:	LN:		Abdomen:	
Overall:			Heart sounds:	Lung sounds:
Documentation				
Radiographs:	Digital	Film		
Digital photos:				
Referred by:				
Recommended follow-up:				

CANINE ORAL DIAGNOSIS, TREATMENT PLAN, AND TREATMENT CHART

M2	M1	P4	P3	P2	P1	C1	I3	I2	I1	I1	I2	I3	C1	P1	P2	P3	P4	M1	M2
110	109	108	107	106	105	104	103	102	101	201	202	203	204	205	206	207	208	209	210

DX · PLN · TX · RT · B · O · P · L · O · B

M3	M2	M1	P4	P3	P2	P1	C1	I3	I2	I1	I1	I2	I3	C1	P1	P2	P3	P4	M1	M2	M3
411	410	409	408	407	406	405	404	403	402	401	301	302	303	304	305	306	307	308	309	310	311

Remarks:

_____

_____

_____

_____

_____

Appendix 3　Feline Dental Chart

Clinic name: _____

Doctor Name: _____　Phone: _____

Date: _____　Fax: _____

Client name: _____　Client #: _____

Patient name: _____　Age: _____ Sex: _____ Breed: _____

Color: _____ Weight: _____ Allergies: _____

Medical alert			
Chief complaint			
Past dental history			
Pertinent history			
Diet			
Home care	Brush	Rinse	Medications
Other			

Initial Exam		
SKULL TYPE	**DENTAL ABNORMALITIES**	**MISC**
Brachycephalic	Ret. deciduous _____	Oral enlargements
Mesocephalic	Missing _____	Pharynx
Dolichocephalic	Supernumerary _____	
Other	Caries _____	TMJ
OCCLUSION	Broken _____	Other
Normal scissors	Discolored _____	
Class I:	Gingival recession _____	
PM shift		
Anterior crossbite	**INDEXES**	
Posterior crossbite	Overall calculus index (CI)	
Rostrally deviated max K9	(0) None	
Base narrow lower canines	(I) Supragingival/w sl. subgingival	
Class II:	(II) Moderate subgingival	
Brachygnathic/over	(III) Abundant supragingival and/or subgingival	
Class III (prognathic/under):	Gingivitis index (GI)	
Level/reverse scissor/	(0) None	
underbite	(I) Mild/no bleeding	
Other:	(II) Moderate/bleeding on probing	
Wry	(III) Severe/spontaneous bleeding	
Occlusal wear		
ICPM		

Physical Exam				
Temperature:	F	Pulse (BPM):		Respiratory rate:
CRT:	LN:	Abdomen:		
Overall:		Heart sounds:		Lung sounds:
Documentation				
Radiographs:	Digital	Film		
Digital photos:				
Referred by:				
Recommended follow-up:				

FELINE ORAL DIAGNOSIS, TREATMENT PLAN, AND DENTAL TREATMENT CHART

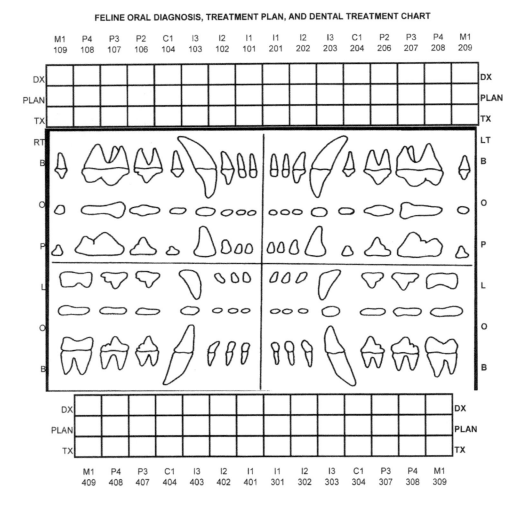

M1	P4	P3	P2	C1	I3	I2	I1	I1	I2	I3	C1	P2	P3	P4	M1
109	108	107	106	104	103	102	101	201	202	203	204	206	207	208	209

DX — DX
PLAN — PLAN
TX — TX
RT — LT
B — B
O — O
P — P
L — L
O — O
B — B
DX — DX
PLAN — PLAN
TX — TX

M1	P4	P3	C1	I3	I2	I1	I1	I2	I3	C1	P3	P4	M1
409	408	407	404	403	402	401	301	302	303	304	307	308	309

Remarks: _____

_____

_____

_____

_____

_____

_____

APPENDICES

Appendix 4   Dental Procedure Estimate

This document lists procedures to be performed on Kodi. *This estimate only approximates the cost of this visit. It does not include any treatments that may be deemed necessary upon examination and commencement of the included treatments.* You are responsible for all fees incurred during this visit included or not in this estimate.

The following is a list of the treatments and/or supplies expected to be required during this visit and their approximate cost.

If you have any questions concerning this estimate, please do not hesitate to ask.

Procedure or dispensed item	Qty	Charge ($)
Preoperative exam		$18.89
Packed cell volume (PCV) with preoperative laboratory tests		$11.01
VetTest Preanesthetic Panel (IDEXX Laboratories, Westbrook, ME; www.idexx.com)		$15.40
Blood collection procedure		$11.35
IV catheter placement and supplies		$25.00
Preanesthesia acepromazine, buprenorphine, and atropine		$12.78
Ketamine and diazepam induction		$35.60
Isoflurane intubation maintenance first 15 minutes		$29.81
Isoflurane intubation maintenance	3	$40.24
Grade 3 periodontal therapy		$84.41
Dental survey x-rays 20–60 lb		$43.90
Tooth extraction – Level 3		$35.00
Tooth extraction – Level 4		$65.00
Dental Nerve Block		$50.00
Metacam 5 mg/mL injectable	0.50	$10.13
Metacam 1.5 mg/mL 100 mL	5	$11.48
Clavamox tabs 375 mg	14	$32.40
Tramadol 50 mg	6	$10.90
Total estimate charges		$543.30

Be assured that the health of Kodi is our highest concern and we will do everything possible to maintain that health. Understand, too, that your signature below indicates that you have reviewed and agree to the terms of this estimate.

Your signature below does not make you responsible for the charges listed above unless performed upon Kodi.

I accept and agree to the terms of this estimate:

_____

John Smith

Appendix 5   Dental Procedure Release Form

555-555-555

Dr. Smith

August 10, 2010

Owner:	Beau Smith	Patient:	Barney
Case no:	1234	Breed:	Beagle
Street:	1234 Any St.	Sex:	NM
City:	Anytown	Age:	5 yr
Phone:	555-123-1234	Color:	Tri-colored

I, the undersigned, do hereby certify that I am the owner (duly authorized agent for the owner) of the animal described above, that I do hereby give <serv-doctor>, his agents, and/or representatives full and complete authority to perform the surgical procedure described as:

☐ Scaling and polishing (remove plaque and tartar) and full series radiographs (a complete set of X-rays are included in the cost of this procedure)
☐ Necessary extractions (after calling for consent)
☐ Necessary extractions (without calling)

and to perform any other procedure that, at his discretion, may be useful to promote the health of the above described pet, and I do hereby and by the presents forever release the said doctor, his agents, or representatives from any and all liability arising from said surgery on said animal. *If we are unable to reach you by phone, the doctor will make the necessary decision for the health of the animal.*

LABORATORY TESTING

In an effort to provide the best possible care for your pet, we are requiring preanesthetic blood screening for all pets undergoing anesthesia. Because we will be using injectable medications, it is important to know if there are any hidden health concerns your pet may have that are not detectable with a physical exam. Our in-house blood work screens for anemia and vital organ health. This information can serve as a baseline for future reference.

Signed _____ Alt. phone #_____

Beau Smith

PAYMENT IS DUE AT THE TIME OF SERVICE.

Appendix 6   Dental Radiograph Template

Feline Radiographs

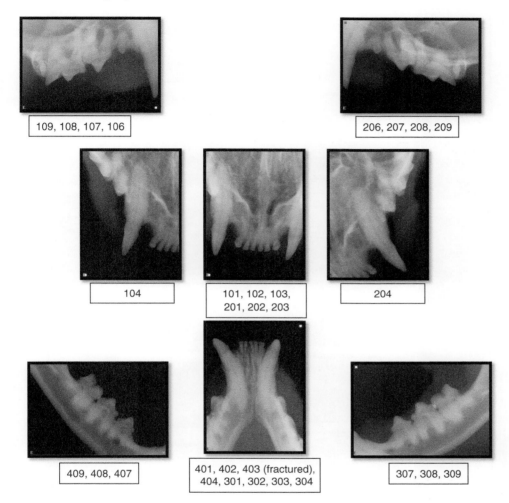

109, 108, 107, 106

206, 207, 208, 209

104

101, 102, 103, 201, 202, 203

204

409, 408, 407

401, 402, 403 (fractured), 404, 301, 302, 303, 304

307, 308, 309

Canine Radiographs

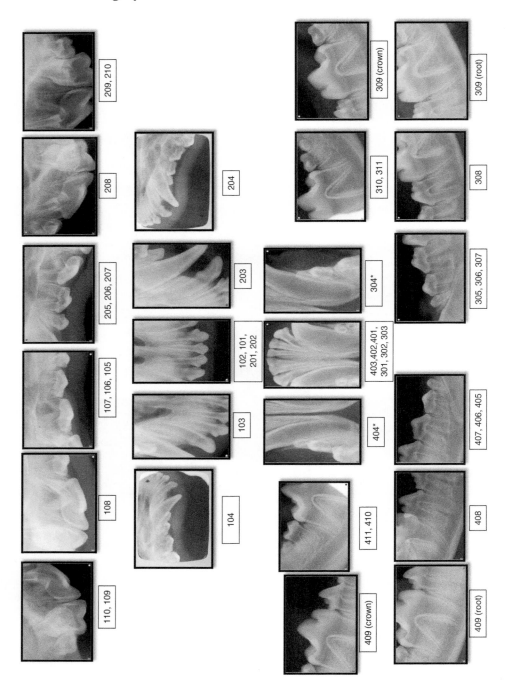

Your LOGO Here

Doctor's Name
Address
Phone Number
Email
Website

Patient: "Roo"
Date: 3/28/19

Dental Procedure Discharge Instructions

Roo had a complete dental prophylaxis today. This includes a full cleaning above and below the gumline using a Piezo ultrasonic scaler. The teeth are then polished to restore the enamel to a smooth surface. The final step of the procedure is to apply a fluoride treatment. A mild sedative/pain reliever is given in the morning to help alleviate any anxiety or discomfort associated with the procedure. An antibiotic is given by injection while under anesthesia if severe infection is found in the oral cavity. Intravenous fluid therapy is administered to maintain circulation, hydration and blood pressures within normal range. The site where the IV catheter is placed must have the hair shaved and cleaned to ensure sterility. Any bruising should dissipate within a few days and the hair will grow back within a few weeks. Any additional shaved areas are for proper placement of our anesthetic monitoring equipment.

Roo had a moderate amount of tartar removed from her teeth. *A full oral exam showed severe periodontal disease which led to bone loss, root infections and tooth mobility. Dental radiographs confirmed the need for removal of ** teeth. Adult dogs have 42 teeth, since she was already missing ** teeth – this leaves her with ** healthy and stable teeth.* Dental radiographs confirmed removal of all tooth root material with no damage to the surrounding bone or teeth. Sutures were placed to encourage tissue healing and the oral cavity was flushed with an antimicrobial solution. This will help prevent any further infection and discomfort to Roo. The rest of her teeth appear normal and healthy. Roo has had pain relievers to make her feel more comfortable and may be groggy while she is on them.

Extractions are sometimes necessary when a tooth or its roots are too infected to save. Frequently the pet seems more active and comfortable once the diseased teeth are removed. Do not become alarmed if you notice some bloody saliva around your pet's mouth, this is normal and will resolve within a few days. You can use a small towel or gauze with warm water to wipe any discharge away from the mouth. *Please call right away if there is any active or profuse bleeding. The underlying bone will take up to a few weeks to heal, so we recommend restricting any chewing on toys, bones, sticks or rocks during this healing period. Also, avoid any tug of war or excessive rough playing during this healing period.*

Regular brushing and cleanings will help maintain Roo's good oral health. Remember, dental disease can be prevented with consistent at-home care. Brushing the teeth, oral gels, oral rinses, dental diets and dental chews will help maintain your pet's good oral health. This is the best way to help prevent periodontal problems in the future.

Medications:

Convenia injection – An injection of an antibiotic was given under the skin today that will provide the appropriate dosing within her system for the next 14 days. (**Antibiotic**)

Buprenorphine Liquid (0.4 mL/syringe) – Give one syringeful by mouth (transmucosally – which means try to get the liquid to the mucosa – inside the cheek, inside the inner lips, or under the tongue) 2–3 times a day until gone. (**Pain Medication**)

Rimadyl 25 mg – Give 1 tablet by mouth TWICE a day until gone. (**Anti Inflammatory**)

Start medications tonight with a small soft meal.

■ Roo's nails were trimmed and ears cleaned while under anesthesia today.

Roo's special instructions are below:

■ Roo can have small amounts of food and water following today's discharge from the hospital. Offering smaller amounts will be easier on your pet's stomach in case they are nauseous from the anesthesia or pain relievers. Since Roo had extractions, please feed canned or softened food for 7 days. (Avoid things that are too hot or too cold. Also stay away from things that are stringy or sticky, as they may get caught in the stitches – Examples: peanut butter, cream cheese, etc.)
■ Any sutures in the oral cavity are absorbable and will dissolve on their own within the next 2 weeks.
■ **Please schedule a recheck in 7–10 days to have the extraction sites evaluated.**
■ Please contact us with any questions or concerns.
■ *Thank you for trusting us with your pet's oral health needs.*
■ Veterinarian: Doctor's Name
■ Technician: Technician's Name

Appendix 8   Discharge Take Home Pictures: Simple Example

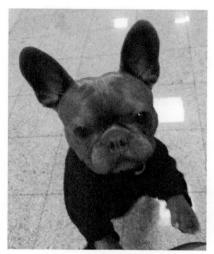

Tsonga's Dental Procedure

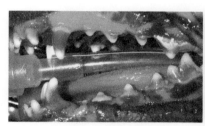

Before cleaning

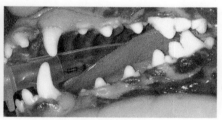

After cleaning

Dental radiographs

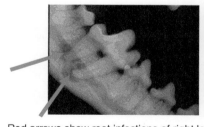

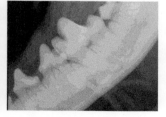

Red arrows show root infections of right lower first molar

Your LOGO Here

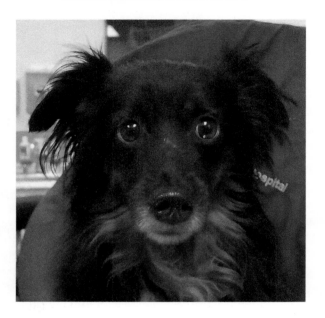

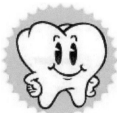

Roo's

Dental

Procedure

3-28-19

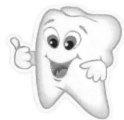

ROO 3/28/2019

Right Side Before

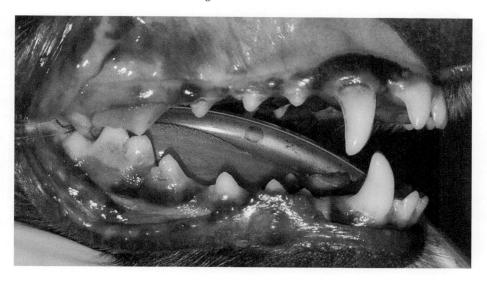

Right Side After

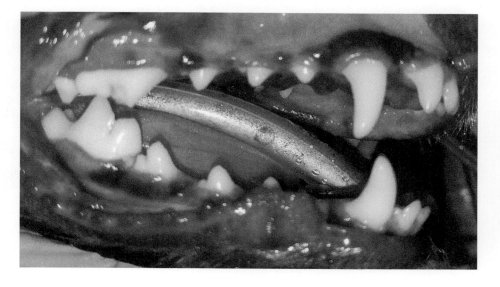

Left Side Before

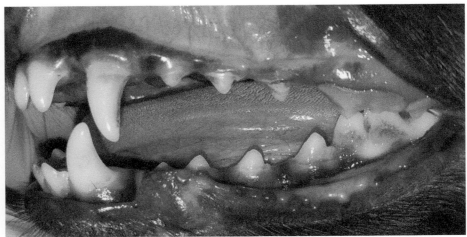

Left Side After

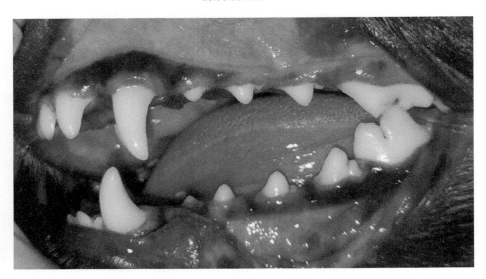

Close ups showing fractures with near pulp exposure

Right Upper Fourth Premolar

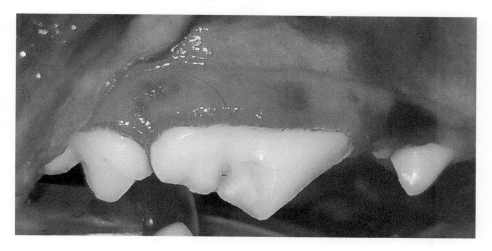

Left Upper Fourth Premolar

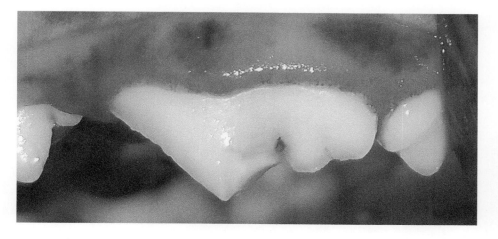

Dental Radiographs

Right Upper Quadrant

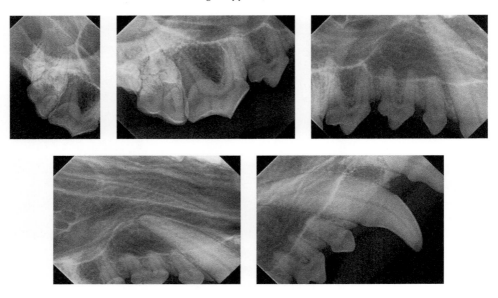

Left Upper Quadrant

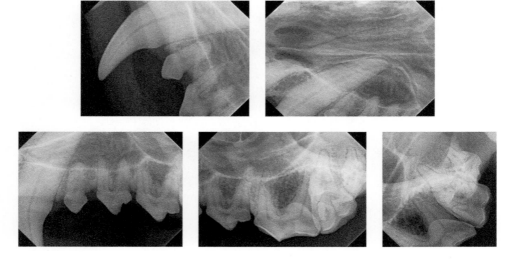

Right Lower Quadrant

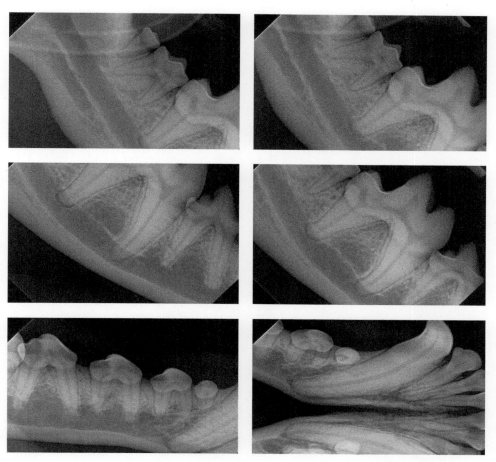

Left Lower Quadrant

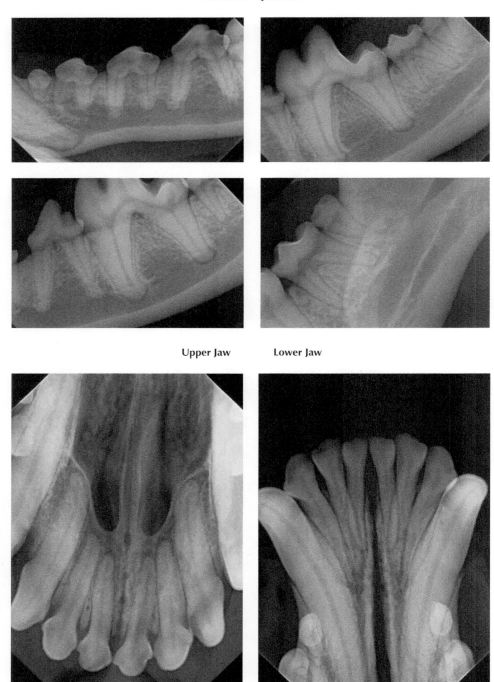

Upper Jaw   **Lower Jaw**

Roo has all 42 of her adult teeth, both upper fourth premolars have fractures with near pulp exposures. The rest of her teeth appear healthy and stable at this time. ☺

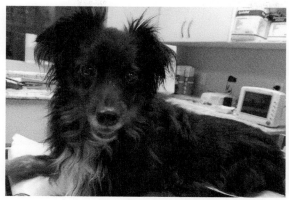

Thank you for trusting us with your fur baby ☺

Index

Page locators in **bold** indicate tables. Page locators in *italics* indicate figures. This index uses letter-by-letter alphabetization.

Small Animal Dental Procedures for Veterinary Technicians and Nurses, Second Edition.
Edited by Jeanne R. Perrone.
© 2021 John Wiley & Sons, Inc. Published 2021 by John Wiley & Sons, Inc.